THE NATURAL WAY SERIES

Increasing numbers of people worldwide are falling victim to illnesses which modern medicine, for all its technical advances, often seems powerless to prevent – and sometimes actually causes. To find cures for these so-called 'diseases of civilization' more and more people are turning to 'natural' medicine for an answer. The *Natural Way* series aims to offer clear, practical and reliable guidance to the safest, gentlest and most effective treatments available – and so to give sufferers and their families the information they need to make their own choices about the most suitable treatments.

Special note from the Publisher

A variety of terms such as 'alternative medicine', 'complementary medicine', 'holistic medicine' and 'unorthodox medicine' are commonly used to describe many of the treatments mentioned in this book but because in practice they all mean much the same the publishers have opted for the single term 'natural' to describe them all. 'Natural' in the context of this series means treatments which are first and foremost gentle, safe and effective and above all avoid the use of toxic drugs or surgery. The treatments described are mostly tried and tested, and many have been proven effective in medical trials, but some have not. Where treatments are interesting and intriguing but speculative at present this has been clearly indicated.

The books in this series are intended for information and guidance only. They are not intended to replace professional advice, and readers are strongly urged to consult an experienced practitioner for a proper diagnosis or assessment before trying any of the treatments outlined.

Other titles in the series

The Natural Way With

Arthritis &
Rheumatism

Pat Young

Series editor
Richard Thomas

Series medical consultants
Dr Peter Albright MD & Dr David Peters MD

Approved by the
AMERICAN HOLISTIC MEDICAL ASSOCIATION
& BRITISH HOLISTIC MEDICAL ASSOCIATION

ELEMENT
Shaftesbury, Dorset ● Rockport, Massachusetts
Brisbane, Queensland

© Pat Young 1995

First published in Great Britain in 1995 by
Element Books Limited
Shaftesbury, Dorset

Published in the USA in 1995 by
Element, Inc.
42 Broadway, Rockport, MA 01966

Published in Australia in 1995 by
Element Books Limited
for Jacaranda Wiley Limited
33 Park Road, Milton, Brisbane 4064

Cover design by Max Fairbrother
Designed and typeset by Linda Reed and Joss Nizan
Printed and bound in Great Britain by
BPC Paperbacks Limited

British Library Cataloguing in Publication
data available

Library of Congress Cataloging in Publication
data available

ISBN 1-85230-629-7

Contents

List of Illustrations

To my dear friend Freddie Phillips, whose father
Francis Phillips died from the consequences of
treatment for rheumatoid arthritis

Acknowledgements

The author wishes to express grateful thanks to the following for permission to draw from their material in the preparation of this book. Individual sources of information are noted in the text and full references appear in Appendix B.

The Arthritis and Rheumatism Council
Arthritis Care
The Consumers' Association (publishers of *Which? Way to Health*)
Little, Brown (publishers of *Overcoming Arthritis*, by Dr Frank Dudley Hart)
Pan Books Ltd (publishers of *Rheumatism and Arthritis*, by Malcolm Jayson and Allan Dixon)
Beaconsfield Publishers Ltd (publishers of *Classical Homoeopathy*, by Dr Margery Blackie, from which the case study on p. 74 is taken

Introduction

About twenty million people are affected in the UK
alone by *some* form of rheumatic disease, and this
statistic is reflected throughout the world. It is the single
biggest cause of disability, seriously affecting about a
third of all sufferers in Britain – that is, between seven
and eight million people.

The term 'rheumatic disease' embraces about 200
different types of arthritis and rheumatism, and of these
the two most common forms are the degenerative
disease *osteoarthritis*, and the inflammatory disease
rheumatoid arthritis. Both affect the joints and, like all
forms of arthritis, can cause intractable pain and severe
disability in their advanced stage.

In spite of the amount of research being done, medical
science has not as yet discovered the cause of
inflammatory arthritis, and consequently there is no cure
for it. Osteoarthritis is caused by wear and tear on the
joints, but it is not yet known why some people are more
susceptible to joint degeneration than others.

While surgery can now offer almost miraculous relief
of pain and disability by replacing diseased joints, drug
therapy for rheumatic disease is beset by the problem
that the risks and side-effects of treatment may outweigh
the benefits. It is no wonder that people afflicted with
rheumatic disease seek relief in the field of natural
therapy, where treatments are gentle and do not have
unpleasant side-effects.

My own interest in natural therapy was aroused when, as editor of *Nursing Mirror*, I led a study tour of the healthcare system in China in 1977. We saw traditional Chinese medicine, mainly acupuncture and herbal medicine, being practised side by side with Western medicine, so that patients were given the benefits of both ancient and modern methods.

It is reassuring to know that Western conventional medicine now acknowledges the value of the so-called non-conventional or natural methods of treatment, and that the two branches of medicine are starting to work together more frequently and with mutual recognition and respect. This can only be to the benefit of patients.

By combining information about treatments that both conventional medicine and natural therapy can offer to those unfortunate people who suffer from some form of rheumatic disease, it is hoped this book will widen the range of choices available to them, and in some small way help to solve their problems.

Pat Young

CHAPTER 1

What are arthritis and rheumatism?

How they differ and who is affected

How often have you heard people say, 'It's just a touch of rheumatism', when their back is aching or their joints are stiff and painful and they don't want to make a fuss about it? The word 'rheumatism' is a convenient generality to use for any aches and pains whose cause we aren't sure of, while the word 'arthritis' sounds much more specific. And that, in fact, is the difference.

Rheumatism is a general term used by lay people to describe any painful condition of what is called the 'musculo-skeletal system': the muscles, tendons, bones, and joints that form the structure of our bodies. *Arthritis*, on the other hand, refers specifically to conditions affecting the joints, either inflammatory, as in rheumatoid arthritis, or degenerative, as in osteoarthritis. The medical term for all the conditions that affect the musculo-skeletal system is 'rheumatic disease'.

There are about 200 different types of rheumatic disease, including several different types of arthritis, and they can afflict people of all ages, from nine months to ninety years old, though some of them attack certain age groups and are more common in one or other of the sexes.

For the sake of accuracy and simplicity, conditions affecting the joints will be grouped here under the heading of 'arthritis', and those affecting the other parts of the musculo-skeletal system under 'rheumatism'.

Arthritis:

Common forms of arthritis

- Rheumatoid arthritis
- Osteoarthritis
- Gout
- Ankylosing spondylitis
- Systemic lupus erythematosus
- Juvenile chronic arthritis
- Psoriatic arthritis
- Reactive arthritis

There are two main types of arthritis: inflammatory and degenerative. In inflammatory arthritis the tissues surrounding the joint become inflamed and swollen, often damaging the joint itself. In degenerative arthritis the cartilage protecting the ends of the bones, and eventually the surfaces of the bones themselves, are worn away either by excessive stress or by the wear and tear of ageing. By far the most common forms of arthritis are rheumatoid arthritis (inflammatory) and osteoarthritis (degenerative).

Rheumatoid arthritis

Rheumatoid arthritis is one of the most common of all diseases. About 1 per cent of the whole world population is likely to develop it at some time or other in their lives, and the risks are two to three times higher for women than for men. It can strike at any age, from nine months to ninety years old, but women often get it during their early childbearing years, between the ages of twenty and thirty, or in their fifties, when they are going through the menopause.

Signs and symptoms

The early signs of rheumatoid arthritis are pain and swelling in the joints, usually of the fingers and wrist but sometimes of the feet, shoulders, elbows, knees, and even the jaw. Often the same joints in both arms or legs, for instance, are affected at the same time. The joints are particularly stiff and painful first thing in the morning. The stiffness usually eases up after about an hour, and wears off during the day, but is likely to return at night. The sufferer often also feels generally unwell and feverish.

Rheumatoid arthritis is an unpredictable disease. It may come on suddenly or develop gradually, last for an indefinite time, and vanish quite unexpectedly, sometimes returning again equally unexpectedly. It also varies in severity. It may be mild and easy to live with, needing no more than the occasional aspirin to control the pain. It may be moderate, with occasional acute active phases, and possible to control with drugs and other methods of physical treatment. It may be severe, causing considerable pain, deforming the joints it attacks, and making the sufferer very disabled.

Fortunately only 10 per cent of all cases of rheumatoid arthritis are severe. The majority – 60 per cent – come in the 'moderate' category, while the remaining 30 per cent of cases are mild.

Osteoarthritis

Osteoarthritis should more correctly be called 'osteoarthrosis' since it is degenerative and long term. The suffix 'itis' indicates inflammation, while the suffix 'osis' signifies a 'chronic' condition. (Chronic means it is degenerative and long term, unlike 'acute' which means immediate and short term.) However although, strictly speaking, the term 'osteoarthritis' is inaccurate, it is the one most often used and the one used in this book.

Like rheumatoid arthritis, osteoarthritis is a very common disease. The UK Arthritis and Rheumatism Council estimates that about five million people in Britain suffer from it, although not all of them necessarily have much pain, the changes in the joints only showing up on X-ray.

It affects older people more than any other age group, as their joints are subject to wear and tear through continual use over many years, and may eventually show signs of degenerating. The usual age of onset is about fifty, but younger people may also be affected, particularly those, like sportspeople, athletes, and dancers, who are very physically active and place a lot of strain on their joints. Osteoarthritis may also follow an injury to a joint. Women are slightly more often affected than men.

Signs and symptoms
Osteoarthritis rarely comes on suddenly. It usually makes itself known gradually as a nagging pain in a joint. The joints most often affected are those that have to bear a person's weight – the hips, knees, sometimes the ankles, and the feet, particularly the joint at the base of the big toe.

Unlike rheumatoid arthritis, osteoarthritis only attacks one joint at a time, and it does not make the sufferer feel ill and feverish. The pain is usually worse after exercise and at the end of the day. The joints of the fingers and at the base of the thumb are frequently affected in women, and small bony growths or nodules may form round the joints at the tips of the fingers. These are called 'Heberden's Nodes', after Dr William

Heberden, a celebrated physician who was George III's doctor and who first described these nodules. The joints of the spine (*vertebrae*) are also vulnerable to osteoarthritis.

The pain and stiffness are usually mild, and the *analgesic* (pain-killing) drug most frequently recommended is *paracetamol*. It is also important to keep the muscles and tendons that support the joint in good trim, so appropriate exercises are beneficial. Swimming is the best form of exercise for osteoarthritics, as the water supports the weight of the body and the affected limbs can be exercised more freely than on dry land.

Osteoarthritis becomes severe if the cartilage protecting the bone ends wears away completely, and the bones start rubbing together. The tissue surrounding the joint gets inflamed by small outgrowths of bone round the joint, making it painful and difficult to move. The pain can be sharp and sudden when the joint is moved, or it can be a deep, nagging ache. The joint may become deformed, causing considerable disability, and this is when replacement with an artificial joint may become necessary.

Gout

Two eminent British rheumatologists, Professor Malcolm Jayson and Dr Allan Dixon, have described gout as a 'snob' disease – because it is more common among the rich, successful, aggressive, and intelligent! They go on to illustrate the point with the story that when the Maoris in New Zealand forsook their traditional diet of fish and vegetables for the Western diet of beef, bread, sugar, and dairy products, they showed an alarming tendency to become overweight, to develop diabetes and coronary disease, and above all to suffer from gout.

The old belief that gout is caused by consuming too much port and pheasant is, however, untrue. It is the result of too much uric acid in the blood forming tiny needle-sharp crystals in the joints – especially the big-toe joint – making them excruciatingly painful. These crystals may also appear under the skin, sometimes in the lobe of the ear, and look like small white pimples.

Foods which increase the amount of uric acid in the blood, such as liver, kidney, and sweetbreads, should be avoided, and meat and alcohol should be taken in moderation as too much of them can also bring on an attack. But although gout is very common, particularly among men, it can be successfully controlled by anti-inflammatory drugs, and damage to the affected joints is unlikely.

Once the inflammation is under control another medicine, such as *allopurinol*, is usually given to keep acid levels low.

Ankylosing spondylitis

This is a form of inflammatory arthritis which mainly affects young men. The word 'ankylosing' means stiffening, and 'spondylitis' means affecting the spinal vertebrae, so someone with ankylosing spondylitis has a stiff and painful back.

Usually it starts in the lower back, where the joints that link the pelvis and spine become inflamed. As the disease advances, the inflammation may spread up the spine, and down to the hip and knee joints. In the early stages, the pain gets noticeably worse at night, but many men find that if it becomes intolerable by the early morning, it can be relieved by getting out of bed and doing exercises, such as touching the toes. Sometimes the eyes become inflamed and bloodshot, and immediate treatment is essential to prevent permanent damage.

Usually the disease runs its course, taking anything from five to twenty years, but in rare cases it gets steadily worse, until the sufferer's back is so stiff he can hardly bend or turn at all. In very severe cases the spine becomes deformed and causes great disability.

Systemic lupus erythematosus

Young women are the main victims of lupus, or SLE, as it is frequently called. It, too, is an inflammatory form of arthritis, and can affect many different parts of the body. The symptoms are very like those of flu: fever, fatigue, and aches and pains in the joints and muscles. Its name reflects some of its symptoms: systemic means spread throughout the body, lupus (the Latin word for wolf) describes the rash on the face which is said to be like a wolf's bite, and erythematosus (from erythema or redness) describes the inflammation on the skin.

Because its symptoms are like those of many other illnesses, it can be difficult to diagnose. It may come and go over many years, and suddenly disappear of its own accord. Exposure to the sun can cause lupus to flare up, and so can pregnancy. But one good thing is that, although the joints are subject to inflammation, it rarely does them any permanent damage.

Juvenile arthritis

It may seem unlikely, but children as well as adults can be affected by arthritis. About one child in every thousand in the UK – and probably throughout the world – is attacked by arthritis, usually between the ages of one and four.

There are three different forms of juvenile arthritis.

● *Pauci-articular arthritis* The most common type, this starts at the age of two or three, lasts for several years, and makes only a few joints swollen and painful. The child doesn't usually feel unwell, but there may be eye problems so it is wise to have regular checks made.

- *Polyarthritis* This can start at any age from a few months onwards, affects many joints, and usually spreads quickly from one joint to another. A child suffering from polyarthritis feels generally feverish and unwell, and may also have a rash.

- *Still's disease* Named after Dr George Frederick Still, who identified it while he was working at the famous Great Ormond Street Hospital for Sick Children in London, it mainly affects children under five, and causes fever, rashes, painful joints, swollen glands, anaemia, and other complications.

Children usually 'grow out of' their arthritis after some years, and go on to lead perfectly normal lives with little damage to their joints. But while they have the disease they need to be helped to lead a normal life too, continuing their schooling and keeping up with their friends. Exercise is very helpful to them – especially swimming.

Psoriatic arthritis

This is the type of arthritis that afflicted the late British television playwright Dennis Potter, and which he depicted so vividly in his serial 'The Singing Detective'.

Psoriasis is a common skin disease affecting about 2 per cent of the UK population, and it is sometimes accompanied by a form of inflammatory arthritis that usually affects the spine or the joints at the ends of the fingers and toes, and sometimes also the knees.

Some people who get psoriatic arthritis severely, like Dennis Potter, may develop very deformed joints, but it is not normally crippling, and most people can cope with it well.

Reactive arthritis

This form of arthritis is also called *Reiter's syndrome*, and sometimes – more correctly – *Brodie's disease*. In 1916 Dr Hans Reiter described the case of a German cavalry officer who developed acute arthritis accompanied by inflamed eyes and a discharging penis, but an Englishman, Sir Benjamin Brodie, had already described the same combination of symptoms in 1818.

The condition can be a reaction to a sexually transmitted infection, and it can also be a reaction to a bowel infection. In both cases the symptoms are unpleasant, with inflammation and ulceration. Inflammation also usually occurs in the joints of the feet and knees, but may affect the spine and the arm.

Rheumatism:

Common forms of rheumatism
- Fibromyalgia
- Neck pain
- Back pain
- Painful shoulder
- Bursitis
- Carpal tunnel syndrome
- Polymyalgia rheumatica

The term 'rheumatism' covers all the aches and pains in what is called the 'soft tissue' or 'connective tissue' of the body: the muscles, tendons, ligaments, and all the fleshy parts that move, link, and support the bones and joints. Pain in the soft tissue can be due to strains and sprains, to overuse, to direct inflammation, to obesity – these are just a few causes of general rheumatic aches and pains. But there are about half a dozen specific rheumatic conditions that are worth discussing as they are so common and so troublesome.

Fibromyalgia

This is a new name for our old friends 'fibrositis' and 'muscular rheumatism'. It means simply pain and tenderness in fibrous tissue, and it is most often felt in the shoulders and neck, but can also occur between the shoulder blades, at the elbows, low in the back, in the hips and in the knees. Someone with fibromyalgia is also likely to feel tired and to lack energy. Research has shown that people who sleep badly are susceptible to fibromyalgia – and who hasn't woken up with a stiff neck after a restless night?

Neck pain

The most common cause of a continuously stiff and painful neck is a condition called 'cervical spondylosis', which is due to wear and tear on the vertebrae and intervertebral discs of the neck. There are seven vertebrae in the neck – the cervical vertebrae – at the top of the twenty-four vertebrae that form the spinal column. In between each pair of vertebrae is a disc of cartilage which acts as a shock absorber: these are called the intervertebral discs. Each disc consists of a central jelly-like core surrounded by a strong layer of fibres.

If the intervertebral disc wears and shrinks, it doesn't keep the vertebrae apart and in an attempt to protect themselves they may grow fringes of bone which press on the roots of the nerves where they join the spinal cord. This causes acute pain in the neck, which may run into the shoulder and down the arm. There may also be tingling and numbness in the fingers.

There are, of course, other causes of neck pain, such as whiplash injuries from car accidents, poor posture, or over-strenuous exercise of the neck muscles as in redecorating a ceiling. Tension headaches can also result from the neck muscles being too tense.

Back pain

About two million people in the UK consult their doctor each year complaining of pain in the lower back, says the Arthritis and Rheumatism Council, and about thirty million working days are lost to the economy each year. Most low back pain is due to straining or tearing the muscles or ligaments of the spine.

Only a small proportion of cases are due to the familiar 'slipped disc'. This happens when the fibre surrounding the soft nucleus of the disc becomes weak and allows the core of the disc to protrude and press on a nerve root. The medical term for this is a 'prolapsed intervertebral disc'.

The spinal vertebrae may also degenerate through wear and tear and grow fringes of bone which press on the nerve roots, causing great pain which may extend down the leg, carried by the sciatic nerve. This is one cause of *sciatica*.

Painful shoulder

The most common cause of pain in the shoulder is inflammation of the tissues supporting the joint: the muscles and tendons. This can be caused by overuse or by injury. Another cause is inflammation of the joint capsule (the tissue directly surrounding and containing the joint). This is very commonly known as 'frozen shoulder', because movement is difficult due to pain and stiffness. The pain and swelling may extend down the arm into the hand.

Bursitis

There are one or more *bursae* next to every joint. There are seventy-eight of them on each side of the body. Some are very small and some as large as 3 inches (75 millimetres) across. Bursae are small bags of tissue which act as cushions or pads between a joint and the muscles and tendons surrounding it. Too much friction will make them rough, painful and inflamed, and full of fluid: this is bursitis. The condition can clear up in a matter of weeks, or it may take as long as a year, but it is what is called 'self-limiting' – that is, it will heal itself in its own time.

Carpal tunnel syndrome

This condition occurs in the wrist, where there is a tunnel – the *carpal tunnel* – through which tendons from the arm pass on their way to the hand. This tunnel is a space rather like the bursae whose lining can become inflamed and swollen and press on the nerves which run beside the tendons through the carpal tunnel. If the swelling gets worse, the forefinger, the middle finger, and sometimes part of the ring finger will feel numb, and the pain may spread right up the neck to the arm. The pain can be particularly severe at night. This syndrome is caused by overuse or by injury, and usually requires a minor operation to take the pressure off the nerves.

Polymyalgia rheumatica

This is a rheumatic condition that affects older people and is at least as common as gout. About one in every hundred people aged over sixty-five is vulnerable, though it may occur from the age of fifty.

The onset is usually sudden, the victim feeling generally off colour, with pains in the neck, back, shoulders, and thighs. Stiffness gets much worse after resting, and is particularly bad in the morning, making it extremely difficult to get out of bed. The shoulders are often so stiff that sufferers can hardly lift their arms or get their hands to their mouths to drink a cup of tea or take the tablets prescribed for them.

Not unnaturally, people suffering from polymyalgia rheumatica feel tired and depressed and very conscious of their advancing age, but usually the condition responds dramatically to a drug called *prednisolone*, and the sufferer feels twenty years younger, with far less pain and stiffness.

The cause of polymyalgia rheumatica is not known, nor why it should sometimes be accompanied by a disease of the arteries called *temporal arteritis*, which can be serious as it may block the arteries in the eyes and brain, leading to blindness or stroke. Here again the drug prednisolone can prevent this complication.

Polymyalgia rheumatica usually lasts for two to three years, and then clears up spontaneously – to the great relief of its victims.

CHAPTER 2

All about your bones and joints

How they work and why they're important

Bones and muscles

The musculo-skeletal system is a marvellous and complex mechanism. To begin with, the skeleton is constructed of 206 bones, and these are covered and moved by 650 skeletal muscles.

The bones of the skeleton (*see figure 1*) are divided into two main groups: the so-called *axial* skeleton, or axis of the body – that is, the bones of the spine and chest or *thorax* (*sternum* and rib cage) and the *appendicular* skeleton – the bones of the limbs that are attached to it. At the top of the spine is the skull, which itself is made up of eight different bones.

There are three kinds of muscle.

- *Skeletal*, which make the body move voluntarily
- *Cardiac*, confined to the heart
- *Smooth*, like those in the gut

The job of the skeletal muscles is to move the bones and joints when the brain tells them to. Figure 2 shows how the muscles move a joint. They do this usually in pairs, one contracting while the other relaxes.

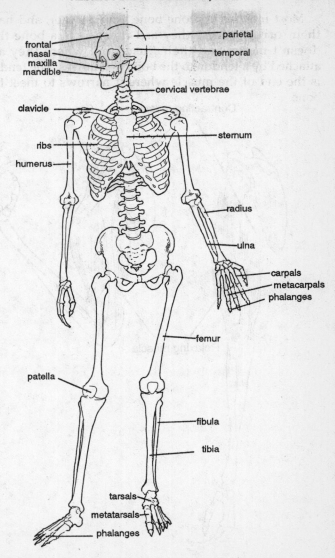

Fig. 1 The human skeleton

Most muscles join one bone with another, and have their 'origin' where they are attached to a bone that doesn't move, and their 'insertion' where they are attached by a tendon to the bone that moves. The tendon is the end of the muscle where it narrows to meet the bone.

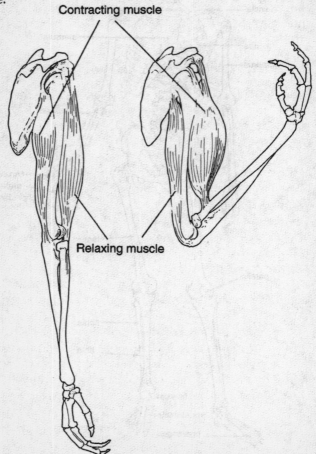

Fig. 2 How muscles move the elbow

Joints

The joints themselves are complicated structures, and there are several different kinds of joint that perform different movements and functions.

One way of classifying the joints is to group them into those that are strong and those that are mobile, with an intermediate group of slightly mobile joints which are strong yet need to be able to move a little.

- *Strong joints* are those between the bones of the skull. When a child is born the eight bones of the skull are not joined together, but as the child grows the bones fuse and the skull becomes rigid.
- *Slightly mobile joints* are those of the spine. The spine is composed of twenty-four bones called *vertebrae* – seven in the neck (the *cervical vertebrae*), twelve behind the chest (*thoracic vertebrae*), five in the lower back (*lumbar vertebrae*), and beneath them a block of bone called the *sacrum*, with a tail-bone called the *coccyx*. The sacrum is joined to the *pelvis* by the *sacro-iliac joints*, and there are joints where other bones, such as the skull and the ribs, meet the spine. Figure 3 is a diagram of the spine.
- *Mobile joints* are those of the limbs and where the limbs join the body, which have to move in different ways in order to perform their individual functions. Some move only in one direction, like hinges, others bend in two directions, or in all directions, and yet others have to bend and rotate, or rotate and fix into position. Finally there are joints which simply move against each other.

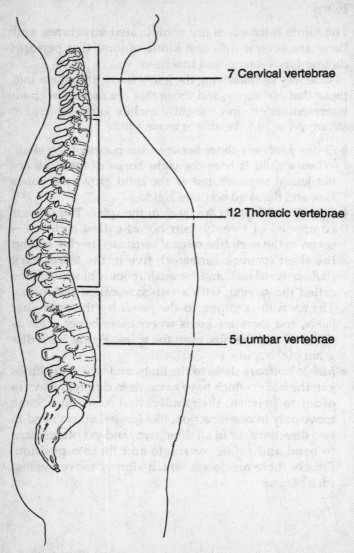

Fig. 3 The spine

Joint types and movement

- *Hinge joint*, moving in one direction – eg finger and elbow
- *Saddle joint*, moving in two directions – eg ankle
- *Ball-and-socket joint*, moving in all directions – eg hip and shoulder
- *Condylar joint*, moving in one direction but also rotating and locking into position – eg knee joint
- *Ellipsoid joint*, with bending and circular movement but no rotation – eg between finger and palm
- *Pivot joint*, with rotation only – eg between head and neck
- *Plane joint*, with flat surfaces moving against each other – eg joint between ribs and thoracic vertebrae.

How joints are constructed

Joints are the point where the ends of two or more bones meet and articulate, or move against each other. Some joints also have to carry the full weight of the body. To do this efficiently they need shock absorbers and lubrication. The *cartilage* that covers the ends of bones, or lies between them like a cushion, acts as a shock absorber, and if it is damaged the bone grows new cartilage to replace it. The lubrication is supplied by a fluid called *synovial fluid*, produced by the *synovial membrane* – the lining of the joint capsule.

The bones that meet in a joint have to be held in place by a bond that is strong yet flexible: this is the *ligament*. Ligaments are strong bands of fibrous tissue connecting one bone to the other and making the joint stable. Each joint has several ligaments. The mobile joints are enclosed within a capsule of fibrous membrane lined with the synovial membrane which delivers a thick sticky fluid (synovial fluid) to lubricate the joint. Figure 4 shows the structure of a normal synovial joint.

When a normal joint is attacked by inflammatory arthritis, such as rheumatoid arthritis, the synovial membrane becomes inflamed, painful and swollen. As the disease advances, fluid and cells leak out of the inflamed membrane and wear away the cartilage on the bone ends. The synovial membrane thickens and spreads into the joint, and eventually not only the cartilage but also the ends of the bones are worn away (*figure 5*). The whole joint then becomes stiff, painful, and possibly deformed as well.

Degenerative arthritis (like osteoarthritis) directly affects the bones themselves, by wear and tear. First the cartilage thins and is worn away, then the bones thicken and spread out at the ends, growing a knobby fringe which protrudes into the joint capsule. The bone ends start to rub against each other, the ligaments are weakened, the synovial membrane is inflamed by friction with the bony outgrowths, and the result is a very painful and unstable joint (*figure 6*).

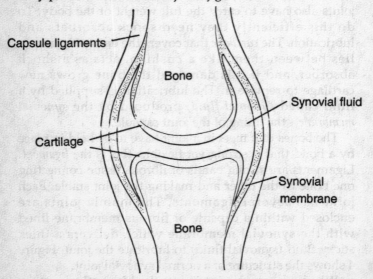

Fig. 4 A normal joint

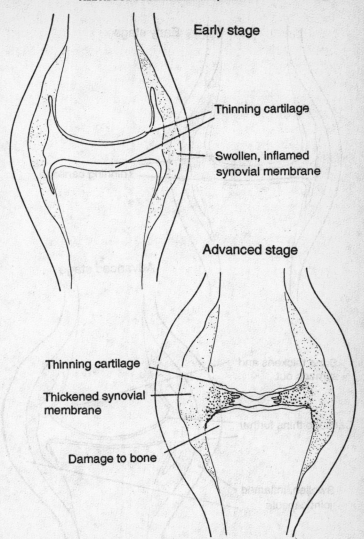

Fig. 5 A joint with rheumatoid arthritis

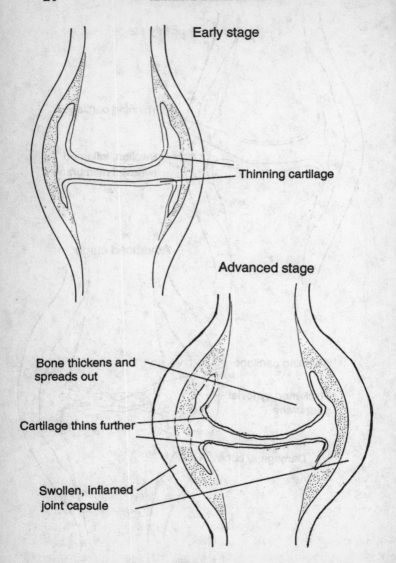

Early stage

Thinning cartilage

Advanced stage

Bone thickens and spreads out

Cartilage thins further

Swollen, inflamed joint capsule

Fig. 6   A joint with osteoarthritis

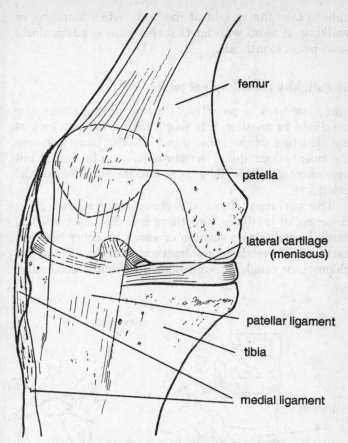

femur

patella

lateral cartilage
(meniscus)

patellar ligament

tibia

medial ligament

Fig. 7 The knee-joint, the most complicated joint in the body

The largest and most complicated synovial joint in the body is the knee, where the large thigh bone (*femur*) joins the two bones of the lower leg (*tibia* and *fibula*), with an extra bone, the *patella*, in front (*see figure 7*). The knee-joint can bend, rotate slightly, and lock into position so that the whole leg is rigid from the hip to the ankle, and able to take the weight of the body when standing or walking. It is no wonder that this joint is particularly susceptible to arthritis.

The slightly mobile spinal joints

Since the back is so often affected by one rheumatic condition or another, it is worth taking a closer look at the structure of the spine (*figure 8*). The joints between the twenty-four spinal vertebrae have to be strong but also move a little, so they come into the 'slightly mobile' category.

The surfaces of the vertebrae have a protective covering of cartilage, and there is a disc (*meniscus*) of cartilage acting as a cushion or shock absorber between each pair of vertebrae: the intervertebral disc. There is a channel, or canal, through which the spinal cord runs,

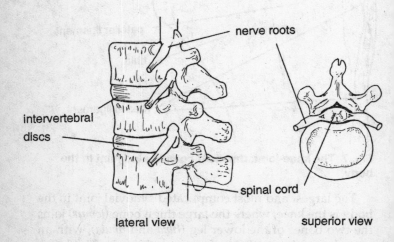

lateral view   superior view

Fig. 8 The bones, joints and nerves of the spine

and the nerves which carry signals from the brain to the rest of the body have their roots in the spinal cord. The nerves emerge from their roots in the cord through small holes in the vertebrae called *foramina* and, if they are damaged by an injury to the spine, part of the body may be paralysed as a result.

The painful condition of the neck known as *cervical spondylosis* is caused by either a disc or a vertebra becoming worn and pressing on a nerve root. Low back pain can also be caused by the fibrous coating of the disc becoming weak and allowing the central core to slip out and press on a nerve root. This is the familiar 'slipped disc', and generally it causes pain in the leg as well as the back.

CHAPTER 3

The causes and effects of arthritis and rheumatism

What they are and how they affect you

There are more than 200 different forms of rheumatic disease and because it would be impossible to describe the causes and effects of all of them in one chapter we will concentrate on the three most common types of arthritis and rheumatism.

● Rheumatoid arthritis (inflammatory arthritis)
● Osteoarthritis (degenerative arthritis)
● Fibromyalgia (muscular rheumatism or *fibrositis*)

Rheumatoid arthritis

Possible causes

No one yet knows exactly what causes rheumatoid arthritis, although a great deal of research is going on in the UK and elsewhere, and several theories have emerged. Perhaps the most plausible theory is that the immune system goes wrong, and the antibodies normally produced to attack infections turn on the body itself and, in a self-destructive process, attack it instead. This process is known as *auto-immune disease*.

It is also thought that a virus may cause rheumatoid arthritis, either attacking the joint lining directly, or infecting normal cells and changing their outer coating so that they become unrecognizable to the *macrophage* cells whose job is to resist and reject unknown and potentially harmful invaders.

This immune process comes into play, for example, in organ transplantation, when it has to be controlled by special drugs (known as *immunosuppressive* drugs) to prevent the donor organ from being rejected. In rheumatoid arthritis, it is believed that the cells in the synovial membrane are changed by a particular kind of virus, called a *retrovirus*, so that they become the target for attack. The retrovirus may lie dormant for years, only being provoked into action by another viral infection.

Another theory is that rheumatoid arthritis can be passed on from one generation to another by a defective *gene* which may render those family members who inherit it susceptible to rheumatoid arthritis, or may influence how severely they get the disease.

It is known that a certain protein described as 'the rheumatoid factor' can be found in the blood of people who get rheumatoid arthritis, and can be identified by a blood test. But as this protein does not appear until the disease has established itself, the test is not very useful for diagnostic purposes.

It is also believed that diet can be a factor, and that eating certain foods – meat and meat products in particular – may make a person more vulnerable. Research has shown that a vegetarian diet may act as a preventive measure, and certainly helps to control symptoms.

As in so many other illnesses, excessive stress can act as a trigger for an attack of rheumatoid arthritis. Many instances have been quoted of how quickly the symptoms can disappear once the source of the stress has been eliminated.

Effects

In inflammatory arthritis the trouble is caused, by definition, by inflammation – not of the joint itself but of the lining and surrounding tissue. The process of inflammation is the body's way of getting to grips with an infection or injury. The blood supply to the affected part increases so that it can deliver more white cells (*leukocytes*) to aid the healing process.

The classical signs of inflammation are heat, redness, swelling, pain, and loss of function. (These are caused by the accelerated flow of blood, and the leakage of healing chemicals in the blood from the small blood vessels into the affected site where they aid healing by neutralizing the cause of the inflammation. The inflammation is prevented from spreading by certain hormones that limit the inflammation to the local site until healing is completed.)

In rheumatoid arthritis the body's healing processes have a difficult and unpredictable enemy to fight. It may attack first one joint and then another, perhaps several at the same time. It may appear and disappear suddenly and unexpectedly, or it may settle in and start to wreak havoc over a long period in the joints it has chosen.

Mild cases   In mild attacks, which constitute about 30 per cent of all cases of rheumatoid arthritis in the UK, the joints of the fingers and wrist are usually the first to become painful and swollen. The pain and stiffness are often worse first thing in the morning, but wear off quite quickly, and the sufferer can keep them at bay with a simple painkiller (such as paracetamol). At this stage only the lining of the joint capsule is inflamed, the inflammation may subside within a few days or weeks, and the joint returns to normal. During this time the sufferer may feel a little feverish, but should feel quite well generally, and probably won't think it is worth while to consult a doctor.

Moderate cases   The majority of cases of rheumatoid arthritis – 60 per cent – come into the 'moderate' category, in which the pain, swelling, and stiffness are more severe and prolonged. The disease may come on suddenly or gradually, and it may affect not only the joints of the fingers and wrist but also those of the feet, shoulders, elbows, knees, and even the jaw.

The joints will typically be particularly stiff and painful first thing in the morning, and though the stiffness will ease up during the day it is likely to return at night. The sufferer often feels generally unwell and feverish, as well as tired, irritable, and depressed.

The pain may skip from one joint to another, affecting first the fingers, then the wrist, then the shoulder, then the ankle or knee. It may affect parallel joints – the same joints in both hands, arms, or legs for instance. It may unexpectedly disappear altogether (go into *remission*), and flare up again equally unexpectedly after an indefinite period of time (*relapse*).

Rheumatoid arthritis is an unpredictable disease, in both the frequency and severity of its attacks. Cold damp weather can make it worse, so a hot dry climate is beneficial.

In these more prolonged attacks of rheumatoid arthritis the inflamed synovial membrane thickens and spreads into the joint space. Excess fluid and cells also leak into the joint and begin to destroy the cartilage covering the bone ends. The ligaments holding the joint stable often become inflamed, and so may the tendons joining the muscles to the bones (*figure 5*). Conventional medical treatment is thus aimed at reducing inflammation and preventing serious damage to the joint.

Inflammation may also occur beneath the skin, and small nodules appear which are tender to the touch. The most usual places for these nodules to manifest themselves are on the forearm, just below the elbow-joint, and in the lower back over the sacrum. *Anaemia* (an iron-deficiency in the blood) may be an added complication.

Severe cases   In the 10 per cent of really severe cases, the inflamed and thickened synovium (lining) wears away not only the cartilage but also the bone ends themselves, so that the joint cannot function properly. The ligaments too are weakened and can no longer hold the bones in place, so the whole joint becomes unstable and deformed. The unfortunate victim suffers great pain and disability, and needs considerable help and support to lead anything like a normal life.

The surgical replacement of such diseased joints with artificial joints can bring miraculous relief of suffering and restore the patient's appearance almost to normal.

Osteoarthritis

Possible causes
Osteoarthritis is even more common than rheumatoid arthritis, affecting 2.5 per cent of adults in the UK. But compared with rheumatoid arthritis, this degenerative disease of joints seems simple and straightforward.

The damage is caused not by inflammation but by wear and tear, either due to excessive use and strain or to the process of ageing. But even after many years of research, no one is yet certain why some people should be more likely to develop osteoarthritis than others.

It is believed that there is a hereditary factor in osteoarthritis, though only some types of the disease, such as that which affects the hands of women in their middle years, are known to run in families. It is also believed that osteoarthritis can occur in a joint that has previously been damaged either by injury or by another form of joint disease.

The ageing process itself has been the subject of a lot of research, and a number of theories about why and how we age have emerged. The biologist Dr Alex Comfort has put forward his theory of 'programmed ageing' – that humans are, like animals, programmed to develop into reproductive creatures, and once their ability to procreate declines their bodies age and eventually die. Others believe that ageing is controlled by the *thymus gland* – the gland that plays an important role in the immune system and is the first organ in the body to start shrinking with age.

It seems more than likely that bones and joints wear out with advancing age – although there is still the amusing story to remember about the ninety-year-old man, seeking advice from his doctor about a painful knee. When the doctor dismissed his patient with the remark: 'What do you expect at your age?', the old man retorted: 'Well, my other knee is the same age, and it's all right!'

All the same, osteoarthritis is regarded as a disease of ageing as it is most common among those who are over fifty years old, although it can start at thirty. In younger people it is likely to follow an injury to the joint, or to be the result of excessive strain on particular joints, as in sport or dancing, or those occupations which involve lifting heavy weights or repeated movements of a particular joint.

Rheumatologists Professor Malcolm Jayson and Dr Allan Dixon, in *Rheumatism and Arthritis*, have referred to 'accelerated breakdown' as another possible cause for osteoarthritis. They point out that wear and tear on a joint can be caused if two parts of a joint don't fit together properly, as often happens in the hip joint. Badly made joints, they say, seem to run in certain families.

There may also be chemical or biological changes in a joint which cause its breakdown, such as when lime salts are deposited in the cartilage. This can cause inflammation, damage to the bone surfaces, and destruction of the lubricating properties of the synovial fluid. Even if the joint recovers, it is likely to break down later on.

Effects

When a joint begins to break down, or degenerate, there may be very little – if any – pain at first. The main symptoms are pain and stiffness, which come on gradually over a period of time – even of years. As there is no inflammation of the joint, the individual feels perfectly well. Only one joint is affected at a time, although it is possible that both hips or knees, being weight-bearing joints, might start to break down simultaneously. The pain is usually worse when the joint is moved and at the end of the day.

The first part of the joint to be affected is the cartilage covering the bone ends. This becomes worn and rough, and may eventually wear away altogether. The bone tries to renew the protective cartilage, but succeeds only in growing little fringes of bone, called *osteophytes*, round its rim, while the surface flattens out (*see figure 6*). As the joint moves the surfaces of the bones start grating together, and the osteophytes irritate the synovial membrane, causing it to become inflamed. The joint becomes swollen and hot as well as stiff and painful.

The joints that most frequently develop osteoarthritis are those that have to bear weight – the hips, knees, and feet, particularly the big-toe joint. Oddly enough, the ankle joint is rarely affected. The complex knee-joint is the one most vulnerable to osteoarthritis.

The non-weight-bearing joints susceptible to osteoarthritis are those of the shoulder, between the collar-bone and shoulder-blade, and of the jaw, in front of the ear. The hands – particularly those of women – are very often affected, and little nodes of bone (called Heberden's Nodes – see Chapter 1) form round the fingertip joints. These nodes, or knobs, are usually painless, but they are a recognizable deformity. If the joint at the base of the thumb is affected, this can be very tiresome as it is involved in almost every movement of the hand.

If osteoarthritis advances to the point where the joint is so stiff and painful it can only be moved with the greatest difficulty, or if it has become quite unstable because of weakened ligaments, surgical replacement with an artificial joint should be considered.

The development of artificial hip joints has been one of the greatest medical advances in recent times, and now knee-joint replacements are even more popular and successful. The relief of constant pain is almost miraculous, and the patient is usually up and moving the limb in two or three days, and walking in two or three weeks.

Fibromyalgia

This is the very common form of rheumatism which used to be known either as 'fibrositis' or as 'muscular rheumatism'. It affects the muscles and tendons, but not the joints, with pain and tenderness, as its name signifies. 'Fibro' refers to fibrous tissue, 'my' to muscles, and 'algia' to pain. It is quite closely connected to ME – *myalgic encephalomyelitis* – the troublesome condition that has only recently been identified, and which is sometimes called 'post-viral fatigue syndrome' because it is believed to follow a virus infection.

The symptoms of both conditions are similar, consisting of aching, stiffness, and tiredness in the muscles, and severe fatigue and lack of energy. In fibromyalgia, these symptoms are thought to be caused by poor sleep.

Recent research in Canada has shown that people suffering from the fibromyalgia syndrome do not sleep deeply enough. There is a distinct pattern to sleep, which begins with about two hours of very deep sleep during which the eyes do not move. There follow several hours of shallow sleep, termed 'rapid eye movement' (REM) sleep, during which the eyes move restlessly and continually.

People who miss the first phase of deep sleep without dreams, and only experience shallow REM sleep with dreams, were shown to be subject to fibromyalgia. They wake tired, with stiff and painful muscles, often of the neck and shoulders.

The fibromyalgia syndrome can be something of a vicious circle, as the muscle pain can prevent deep, restorative sleep and perpetuate the whole problem of poor sleep leading to pain, stiffness, and fatigue. Depression is likely to follow.

Doctors may prescribe drugs for this self-perpetuating condition, but the only real solution is determined self-help.

CHAPTER 4

How to help yourself

Tips and guidelines for self-management and control

There are three main ways in which people suffering from arthritis or rheumatism can help themselves. They are:

- The right diet
- A combination of rest and exercise
- Mental attitude

What is the right diet?

Dietary advice for the gouty person

- Avoid foods containing purine, for example liver, kidneys, sweetbreads, brains, meat extracts, fish roes, sardines, anchovies, whitebait.
- Drink 5 or 6 pints (3 to 3.5 litres) of fluid a day, including water, tea, coffee and fruit juice.
- Drink alcohol only in moderation.

The only form of arthritis that requires a special diet is gout, because it is caused by an excess of uric acid in the blood, and someone who is susceptible to gout must obviously avoid eating the foods that will increase the level of urate, such as liver, kidneys, and sweetbreads. Losing weight will also help to decrease urate levels, and alcoholic drinks should be taken in moderation, as they can trigger off an attack.

Sufferers from other forms of arthritis will be helped by a low-fat diet – ie one that cuts down on meat and dairy products – but if meat is cut out altogether they must be sure to compensate with other protein-rich foods, such as fish, rice, nuts, and eggs. Oily fish, such as herring and mackerel, are particularly good for arthritics as it has been proved that certain kinds of oil in the diet can help to reduce inflammation. Food supplements such as cod liver oil and evening primrose oil are certainly beneficial – but they have to be taken continuously and for a long time to give real benefit.

Claims have been made for the benefits to arthritics of a number of different foods, including honey, garlic, royal jelly, ginseng, and cider vinegar, but none of these claims has been proved. Some people say that extract of New Zealand green-lipped mussel has helped their arthritis, but research studies have not confirmed its benefits.

A weight-reducing diet will benefit any arthritic person who is overweight, as it will lessen the burden the painful joints have to carry, and make getting about easier. This generally means eating smaller quantities, as your body needs less food if it is burning up less energy than it used to, but sticking to a healthy balanced diet will also help to keep you generally fit. This means eating:

● Only a little sugar, butter, margarine, and animal fat
● Moderate amounts of lean meat, poultry, fish, milk, oil, cheese, yoghurt, peas and beans (pulses), nuts, and eggs
● Plenty of wholemeal bread, cereals, potatoes, fresh fruit and vegetables

Don't forget that milk provides the calcium that strengthens bones, so don't cut your milk intake down too much.

Can rheumatoid arthritis be caused by a food intolerance?

A good deal of research is going on to find out if certain foods may provoke arthritis. That rheumatoid arthritis can be caused by a reaction to food, in the same way as migraine or asthma or some skin diseases, is a persuasive theory. The only way to find out is to go on an 'exclusion' diet – that is, to cut the basic food intake down to a minimum and then to introduce one additional food a day and watch carefully for any adverse reactions. If symptoms of rheumatoid arthritis appear after eating certain foods, they can be excluded from the diet in future. An exclusion diet should only be undertaken under the supervision of a doctor or dietitian, however, as it is important to be sure that nutrition is adequately maintained.

Research into dietary factors is concentrating on rheumatoid arthritis. It is unlikely that osteoarthritis and other forms of the disease (apart from gout) have any links with diet.

Rest and exercise

When joints are very inflamed and painful, it is important to rest them so as not to aggravate the inflammation by movement. But it is equally important to keep the joints mobile and the muscles strong by exercising them. So in arthritis a delicate balance has to be struck between rest and exercise.

Rest

In an acute attack of inflammatory arthritis, rest is essential to give the inflammation a chance to subside, which it won't do if the joints affected are being constantly moved. Splints are sometimes necessary to keep joints, such as those in the hand and wrist, absolutely still. They can be bought at a local chemist, or supplied by the local hospital out-patient department: your family doctor will advise you how to get one. Complete bed-rest may be necessary if the inflammation is widespread.

Never forget that joints which stay in one position for any length of time will stiffen up, and it will be difficult to get them to move again. For example, placing a supporting pillow beneath painful knees when you are resting in bed is asking for trouble: the joints will stiffen into a bent position and may be extremely difficult to straighten again. So lie flat in bed with your limbs as straight as possible to prevent them stiffening into one position. But move your affected joints gently several times a day while you are resting them in order to keep them mobile.

When your inflammation has subsided and you are able to get up and about again, it is a good idea still to have a period of rest every morning and afternoon. And exercise your joints gently after you have had a bath or a shower, when they are warm and easier to move. Put them through their natural range of movement until they become painful – but try and move the pain threshold a little further on each day.

Exercise
Doing exercises regularly each day can be boring and requires quite a lot of self-discipline, so it may help to remember what are the aims of regular exercise for an arthritic person. They are:

● To keep your affected joints mobile
● To strengthen your muscles
● To keep you generally fit and healthy

If you sit or lie about all day without taking any exercise, your joints will stiffen up, your muscles will get weak, you will find moving about requires more and more effort, and you will feel generally tired and frustrated. But if you work out and stick to a daily exercise regime, your joints will improve their range of movement, the pain will become less, you will prevent permanent stiffness, and you will feel much better in yourself.

'Operation de-freeze'   An eminent rheumatologist, Dr Frank Dudley Hart, in *Overcoming Arthritis*, has described the daily exercise regime for arthritics as 'operation de-freeze'. By this he means keeping the joints from becoming stiff and restricted, and he recommends doing exercises every morning and evening, preferably after a hot bath or shower.

Physiotherapists, also known as physical therapists, are expert at devising suitable exercise regimes for rheumatoid patients, so you would be wise to consult a local practitioner or ask your doctor to refer you to the relevant department at your local hospital, where a therapist will teach you what exercises to do at home.

Exercises for joint movement   These will involve putting the joints through their normal range of movement as far as the pain permits: bending and straightening a hinge joint like the elbow or the knee, rotating a ball-and-socket joint like the shoulder or hip. You may find it easier to exercise the spine, hips, knees and feet while sitting or lying down, so that your joints are not carrying your weight. Exercising the joints in water is particularly helpful, provided the water is reasonably warm, as it supports your weight and makes joint movement much easier.

Exercises for muscle strengthening   These simply make your muscles work hard in order to improve their 'tone' or strength, so that they don't atrophy from disuse. Don't forget that 'if you don't use it, you lose it'!

Isometric exercises – active exercises against resistance – are particularly useful in improving muscle tone. The therapist will devise a programme of graded exercises for you to work through that will restore the normal functions of the body.

If you do not have access to a therapist or a physical therapy department, you can usually get advice about exercise regimes for arthritic patients from the national organization for therapists. In Britain this is the Chartered Society of Physiotherapy at 14 Bedford Row, London WC1R 4ED.

Exercise for general fitness   The best form of exercise for people suffering from any rheumatic disease is swimming, as it exercises the whole body while it is supported by the water. Half an hour's brisk walk every day is another excellent form of exercise, and so is cycling. Regular exercise in the fresh air will make you generally more healthy and able to cope with the pain and other problems that arthritis inevitably brings.

Mental attitude

The constant pain from arthritis can be very debilitating. Sleep may well be disturbed, and the sufferer wakes tired, irritable and depressed, and less able to cope with problems. Stress, as we know, can act as a trigger for rheumatoid arthritis, so it goes without saying that the stress of suffering from a painful rheumatic disease is bound to make it worse. So what can be done to lessen and overcome the stress?

There are natural methods of treating the mind, as well as the body, as you will read in Chapter 9, but here it is worth emphasizing the value of simple relaxation techniques, such as the following.

- Find a quiet room where you can lie down comfortably, flat on your back for about twenty minutes.
- Empty your mind of all troublesome thoughts, and imagine yourself in a particularly beautiful place – in the countryside or on a peaceful beach. Imagine the sounds of birds and insects, or of seagulls and the sea – sounds that help to create a really tranquil scene in your mind.
- Taking each part of your body – first each foot, then the whole leg, then each hand and arm, and so on right up to your face and head – first contract the muscles, then relax them completely so that they are quite inert. By the time you have finished, your whole body will feel heavy and immovable, and if someone lifted your arm, for instance, it would flop back on to the floor.
- Lie like that for about five minutes, still imagining your ideal tranquil scene and hearing its sounds, and then bring yourself slowly back to reality. Don't hurry: move each part of your body gently, and when you are ready to get up you will be amazed how relaxed you feel, in both mind and body. Your pain should be less too.

The British Holistic Medical Association publishes audiotapes for relaxation as part of its *Tapes for Health* series. See Appendix A for their address and also details of natural health organizations in other countries.

Some solutions for practical problems
It always helps to be practical when problems abound, and there are a number of ways in which you can help yourself in your daily life.

For example, you may need a really comfortable chair, one that supports your back, and is of the right height to make sitting down and getting up again easy.

Why not treat yourself to a new chair with a spring-assisted or motorized seat, with padded arm-rests of the right height, and with a back-rest shaped to the contours of your spine? A well-designed chair can make all the difference to your daily comfort.

You may find climbing stairs is becoming a problem. If you don't want all the upheaval of moving to a flat or a bungalow, or of installing a ground-floor toilet in your own house, why not consider installing a stair-lift? A range of stair- or chair-lifts is usually on display at disabled living centres in most major cities, and some are advertised in magazines and local newspapers. (If you have difficulty in getting information, the local department of your social services or community occupational therapy unit should be able to help. Your family doctor can usually arrange for an assessment of your special needs at any of these places.)

You may be a keen gardener, but find that you are having difficulty in carrying on with the regular jobs that have to be done if your garden is not to turn into a jungle. If bending down to tend your flower beds is a problem, have you thought of building raised beds that you could reach easily sitting on a stool? And have you thought of looking for tools and other equipment specially designed for gardeners with some disability? In Britain the Arthritis and Rheumatism Council (ARC) publishes an excellent booklet *Gardening with Arthritis* which is full of useful information and suggestions for making your gardening life easier. The address is in Appendix A.

You may have found that your arthritis has interfered with your ability to drive, but you will naturally want to carry on driving as long as you can. Again, the UK Arthritis and Rheumatism Council produces an information leaflet *Driving and Your Arthritis* which tells you about the special adaptations to your car that would help you, and gives, for British readers, the addresses of useful organizations such as the Disablement Information and Advice Line (DIAL UK), the Mobility Advice and Vehicle Information Service (MAVIS), the Disabled Drivers' Association and others.

Arthritis and rheumatism organizations in most Western countries publish a wide range of leaflets and booklets to help arthritic people cope with their problems and understand their particular disease. Some, like the Arthritis and Rheumatism Council in the UK, also fund research projects and support research units in hospitals and universities, fund the appointment of professors and lecturers in rheumatology in medical schools, and support bursaries and scholarships to help the paramedical professions develop their knowledge and experience in treating sufferers from rheumatic disease. Their addresses are given in Appendix A.

Another voluntary organization in the UK well worth contacting is Arthritis Care (see Appendix A for the address). It provides information, for people of all ages suffering from arthritis or rheumatism, by mail and by telephone, and produces a range of helpful publications. It has over 500 branches throughout Britain which hold regular meetings for members to share information, organize activities, and help and support each other. In addition it runs specially equipped holiday centres, self-catering holiday units, and a residential home for those who are very disabled.

Finding solutions to the practical difficulties of daily life can help develop a better state of mind, and in the next chapter we will look at aids to daily living for the arthritic person at home.

CHAPTER 5

Aids to daily living
Practical hints and helpful gadgets

Because arthritis can make joints painful, stiff, difficult to use, and sometimes permanently deformed, the normal movements you make in daily living – washing, going to the toilet, shaving, dressing, cooking, doing housework, shopping – can easily become a problem.

For example, arthritis in the hands can make it difficult to grip and hold things, while arthritis in the spine can make bending down a struggle. One way to help yourself in this predicament is to change the way you do things. Another is to look for gadgets that will make doing things easier.

In Britain the Arthritis and Rheumatism Council publishes a handbook for patients *Your Home and your Rheumatism* which is full of useful tips for people who are handicapped by arthritis and rheumatism. Here are just a few of them.

Around the house

To save you bending
If your electric points are at floor level, have them raised to about waist level, so that you have to bend as little as possible to reach the switch. Attach a wire basket to your letter box so that you don't have to bend down to pick up your mail from the door-mat.

To save you slipping
Make sure your floor coverings have no tears in them which might trip you up. Loose rugs which may slip or wrinkle up can be attached to the carpet by a special adhesive tape. Bright lighting will help you to see any small obstacles that might otherwise prove a hazard.

Opening doors
An ordinary door-knob may be difficult for an arthritic hand to grasp, so have these replaced with lever-type handles, which you can operate with your forearm or elbow if necessary. Keys can be difficult to turn, so try putting a skewer through the hole in the end of a mortice lock key to act as a lever. 'Yale' lock keys can be modified to give you a better grip when turning them – ask your local locksmith.

Climbing stairs
It is a good idea to have something to hold on to on both sides of the stairs. A hand-rail on the wall opposite the banister will give you extra security and support. Short flights of steps can be covered by a gently sloping ramp. Stairs should also be well lit, and stair carpets securely fixed so that you cannot trip and fall. Stair-lifts can also be installed, as mentioned in Chapter 4.

In the bathroom
Lever taps can be fitted to your bath and wash-hand basin to make them easier to turn. A hand-rail beside the bath will help with getting in and out, and a non-slip mat in the bath will make it safer. If you can't sit right down in the bath, try using a bath-seat which rests on the sides of the bath and allows you to sit in the water at a comfortable height. A shower, of course, is easier to use, so it's worth considering having one fitted if you haven't already got one.

Using the toilet

If your toilet seat is too low, there are raised seats which can be placed on top of the ordinary toilet seat, and removed when other people want to use the toilet. You may need extra support to help you sit on the toilet, and there is a very useful folding frame which incorporates a raised seat which is portable and can be easily transported. Someone who has to use a wheelchair will need doors on the bathroom and toilet wide enough to allow the wheelchair through, and solid handrails round the toilet. You should get professional advice from an occupational therapist about this.

In the kitchen

It is helpful if all your working surfaces are at the right height to suit you, and all the same height and close together, so that you can slide pots, pans, dishes and so on along without having to grasp and lift them. If your knees or hips are painful, get a high stool – with a back support, if possible – so that you don't have to stand all the time.

Levers can be fitted to your sink taps, and it's worth contacting your local gas or electricity supplier to find out what modified taps they make available on cookers and other kitchen equipment for disabled people.

Shelves within easy reach, cupboards with sliding doors, and lightweight pots and pans will make life easier, and there is a wide range of kitchen gadgets, from tin-openers to potato-peelers, specially designed for people with problem hands.

Eating and drinking

If your grip is poor, you will find it safer to hold cups, glasses, plates and so on with both hands rather than just one. Padding the handles of knives, forks, and spoons will make them easier to hold, and insulated lightweight mugs should be used for drinking hot liquids. There is a wide range of cutlery designed for disabled people, details of which you can get from your nearest disabled living centre or, in the UK, from the Disabled Living Foundation. (Addresses of useful organizations are given in Appendix A at the end of the book.)

Getting dressed

The simple movements you have performed every day of your life – like bending down to put on your socks or stockings – can become almost impossible for someone with painful joints. But a simple gadget called a dressing stick can solve an awful lot of problems. This is a stick with a hook at one end, with which you can pull clothes on, and a rubber tip at the other end, which you can use to push clothes off over your head, for example. You could adapt an old walking stick for this purpose.

Buttons can be difficult to do up, and 'Velcro' fastenings are a boon on clothes. You can also choose clothing which is easy to put on and take off, such as slip-on shoes instead of lace-ups. Dresses and underclothes, such as bras, which fasten in front are easier to wear too. Most countries have national organizations for the disabled that will give practical advice about any problems related to clothing, and about aids for dressing and undressing. In the UK, the Disabled Living Foundation has a special clothing adviser.

Furniture

Perhaps the most important piece of furniture for a sufferer from any form of arthritis or rheumatism is an armchair, as mentioned in the previous chapter. It is well worth a painstaking search to find the one that gives the best support to the body, and that is easy to sit down in and get up from. It is possible to have a chair made to your own measurements and requirements, and although this may be expensive, it will be a good investment for your future comfort, and it can be regarded as your own special chair.

It is important to have tables of the right height for eating or working at, and an adjustable table that tilts to the angle you require can be useful. Use a book-rest if your hands give you trouble. If you find it difficult to write with a slim pen or pencil, try wrapping a piece of foam rubber round it to make it easier to hold. And if you should drop your pen on the floor, or want to reach a book on a high shelf, a pair of tongs can be just what you need. These too are specially designed for people with hand disabilities.

Where to go for advice

The professional person best qualified to give advice about aids to daily living for people with arthritis is the occupational therapist. In most countries, they work both in hospitals and in the community, attached to the local department of social services. If you have had a spell in hospital with your arthritis, and are likely to have some sort of functional problem in coping when you are discharged, the hospital occupational therapist should assess your abilities, perhaps visit your home to see what aids and adaptations you may need, arrange for them to be provided for you, and teach you how to use them and how to cope generally. Many hospitals have rehabilitation units with model kitchens and bathrooms where patients with a residual disability can be shown the gadgets that are available and be taught how to use them.

If your arthritis is not bad enough for hospital treatment, but gives you problems in coping at home, your family doctor can refer you to the local social services department and ask the occupational therapist to assess your needs and provide equipment and support.

UK readers can also go direct to the social services department to ask for help, as under the new Community Care Act they are responsible for providing assistance to those who need it. A word of warning, however. The amount of money available for community care varies from one local authority to another, and thus the 'package of care' each can offer to those in need in its area also varies in quality and extent.

Fortunately there are also many voluntary and charitable organizations in most countries which provide help, both generally and in specific fields. In Britain, as well as ARC and Arthritis Care, the voluntary organizations which will always help if they can include the British Red Cross Society, the Women's Royal Voluntary Service, Age Concern and the Citizens' Advice Bureau. All of them have local branches all over the country, and offer a wide variety of services, both advisory and practical.

In the specialized field of aids for the disabled, which of course includes aids for arthritis sufferers, the information service of the Disabled Living Foundation is pre-eminent in the UK. They can tell you about the most up-to-date aids available and how to obtain them, and give advice on such subjects as clothing, working in the kitchen, and incontinence equipment.

There are also disabled living centres (sometimes existing under a different name) in most leading towns and cities, whose addresses can be obtained from your local telephone directory or from the local social services department.

Using your ingenuity

There is nothing likely to give a better boost to your morale, however, than finding your own solutions to your problems. Having to overcome a disability provides an incentive and a challenge, and you will get a good deal of satisfaction from using your own ingenuity to help yourself. And you will certainly earn the respect of your family and friends!

CHAPTER 6

Conventional treatment

What your doctor is likely to say and do

Because there is no cure for either inflammatory or degenerative arthritis, conventional medical practitioners have to concentrate on alleviating the symptoms of pain and stiffness, reducing inflammation, attempting to prevent deformity and instability of the joint, and by replacing joints which have become too stiff, painful, and deformed for use. They do this by three broad categories of treatment.

- Drug therapy
- Physical therapy
- Surgery

Drug therapy

Practically every drug is toxic to some extent and has adverse side-effects, and the drugs used to treat arthritis are no exception. A careful balance has to be kept between the benefits of a drug and its risks, so that the patient taking it does not suffer more from the side-effects of the drug than from the disease it is being used to treat.

Painkillers
When either rheumatoid or osteoarthritis is mild and in its early stages, a drug to control the pain is all that is

needed. For many years *aspirin* has been the drug of choice, because it also reduces inflammation, but if it is taken in large doses it can cause stomach upsets, bleeding and ulceration, or wheezing and rashes. Because of this *paracetamol* is nowadays usually recommended as the best analgesic (painkiller) for mild arthritis, since it has no side-effects unless it is taken in overdose, when it is toxic to the liver.

Anti-inflammatory drugs

Case history

Mrs Evans, aged fifty-two, consulted her doctor about pain in her hands, shoulders and knees, which was acute at times and kept her awake at night. She was also stiff first thing in the morning. Her doctor looked at her hands and saw that her knuckles were very red and swollen and obviously painful. He asked her if she was feeling well but she told him she felt feverish and under the weather.

He diagnosed rheumatoid arthritis and prescribed an anti-inflammatory drug called *indomethacin*, asking her to let him know how she got on with it. She visited him again in a couple of weeks complaining of headaches and dizziness, which he knew could be side-effects, so he switched her to a less powerful anti-inflammatory drug called *naproxen*. She got on much better with it, and her arthritis improved steadily.

The group of drugs called 'non-steroidal anti-inflammatory drugs' (NSAIDs) has become very popular in treating rheumatoid and other inflammatory types of arthritis, as well as advanced osteoarthritis. These drugs are effective because they both control pain and reduce

.nflammation – an ideal combination for treating arthritis and rheumatism. However, they can produce adverse side-effects in the elderly (who are generally more sensitive to drugs) and in anyone with an allergic disease such as asthma, and they should also be used with caution in anyone who is pregnant or who suffers from stomach ulcers, kidney or liver disorders.

There are many different NSAIDs, with similar properties but with varying side-effects. As patients may respond to one NSAID but have problems with another, a doctor may have to try several before finding the right one.

Second-line drugs
If the pain, stiffness, and inflammation of rheumatoid arthritis do not respond to NSAIDs, there are several 'second-line' drugs that can be tried which produce remissions of the disease after two or three months. They have to be used with great care, however, as their side-effects can be severe.

Gold Gold has been used to treat arthritis for many years, but if used indiscriminately its effects can be disastrous. It is now prescribed only in small dosages, and its effects are closely monitored by regular blood and urine tests. It can affect the kidneys and the blood, but the skin is most vulnerable, and if any rash or itching develops it must be stopped immediately. If strict precautions are taken, it is quite safe and can be very effective.

Anti-malarial drugs Two drugs that were developed for treating malaria, *chloroquine* and *hydroxychloroquine*, have also been used successfully for many years to treat rheumatoid arthritis and systemic lupus erythematosus (SLE), but their side-effects can produce eye problems such as *retinopathy*. Regular eye-checks should be made while a patient is taking them, though the risk to the eyes should be small provided the dosage is also small and the course of treatment limited to two years.

Penicillamine This is a relation of penicillin but not an antibiotic. Like gold, it must be used with caution as its side-effects are similar, and it also suppresses bone-marrow. Consequently regular blood and urine tests are essential to monitor its effects. It can actually *cause* SLE so should *never* be used to treat this condition. Rheumatoid arthritis does not usually respond until six to twelve weeks after a course has started, and the drug is usually only prescribed when the disease is advanced.

Immunosuppressants These include *azathioprine*, *chlorambucil* and *methotrexate* and are useful if a patient does not respond to any of the drugs already mentioned. They can produce nausea, vomiting and diarrhoea, as well as *herpes zoster* (shingles), and careful monitoring is necessary.

Sulphasalazine This has also been found useful in the treatment of rheumatoid arthritis, although it was originally used for *ulcerative colitis*. Its side-effects include rashes, stomach upsets and blood disorders, so frequent blood tests are essential.

Steroids
Steroids were once regarded as something of a 'miracle cure' for most rheumatic conditions, but their side-effects are no longer considered acceptable so they are prescribed with great care. They can cause the well-known 'moon face', as well as diabetes, cataract, heart failure, peripheral vascular disease, osteoporosis, peptic ulceration and thinning of the skin.

The original steroid, *cortisone*, is now no longer used, but one of its derivatives, *prednisolone*, can have a dramatic effect if prescribed judiciously, and is often used to treat SLE and *polymyalgia rheumatica*. In severe cases it can be started in large doses and gradually tapered off to the essential minimum, with remarkable success. Cortico-steroid drugs can be injected directly into painful joints and soft tissue to reduce inflammation.

Case history

Mrs Gibson, a lady of seventy-eight, woke up one morning with a dreadful headache and pains in her arms, shoulders, neck, back and legs. Her shoulders were so stiff that she couldn't even raise her arms to lift a much-needed cup of tea to her lips. She felt so poorly that her husband made her stay in bed and telephoned the doctor, who came round later that morning.

The doctor made a careful physical examination, took some blood for a blood test, told them he suspected she had a rheumatic condition called 'polymyalgia rheumatica', and gave her a prescription for prednisolone. He said he would call in next day with the results of the blood test, and told Mr Gibson to phone him immediately if his wife's headache got worse.

When he called next day he said the blood test confirmed his diagnosis of polymyalgia rheumatica, and that her headache was the result of *temporal arteritis*, a condition that often accompanies polymyalgia and can put the eyesight at risk.

Fortunately the prednisolone had a dramatic effect. Mrs Gibson's headache improved steadily and so did her aching limbs. Soon she was able to get up and about again and go to her doctor's surgery for regular check-ups.

Drugs for gout

Gout is one of the most painful forms of rheumatic disease, and now happily one of the easiest both to treat and to prevent. In its acute phase the NSAID *indomethacin* is usually the drug of choice to reduce pain and inflammation, as it can be tolerated well in high dosage over a short course of treatment. *Colchicine* is an alternative, but it has unpleasant side-effects (nausea, vomiting, diarrhoea and abdominal pain), and in high doses it can be toxic.

Long-term treatment to prevent recurring attacks is with *allopurinol*, a widely used, well-tolerated and effective drug that controls the formation of uric acid.

Physical therapy

Physiotherapy (physical therapy) and occupational therapy are the two physical methods of treatment frequently employed for arthritis. Physiotherapists and occupational therapists often work together in hospital departments of rehabilitation, the physiotherapists assessing the degree of stiffness in the joints, devising individual programmes of exercises to improve their mobility, and relieving pain and stiffness with other methods of treatment such as wax baths and electrotherapy.

The occupational therapists assess the patients' degree of disability as it affects coping with the activities of daily living, teach different ways of performing daily tasks, and demonstrate and provide specially designed gadgets and equipment which will make life easier.

Physiotherapists and occupational therapists also work in the community, treating patients in their own homes.

Physiotherapy for arthritis and rheumatism

The physiotherapist sees patients either in the hospital

ward or in the outpatient department first to assess their condition and then to recommend an individual treatment programme for each patient. Treatment for arthritis is likely to consist of the following methods.

Exercises will be given to mobilize stiff joints and to strengthen muscles which may have become weak from disuse. They may be taught individually or in groups, and if the hospital has a hydrotherapy pool they may be given in water, as the warmth and support of the water encourages easier movement and relaxes joints and muscles.

Electrotherapy: various types of electrical treatments, including short-wave diathermy, interferential and ultrasound therapy, are given to provide gentle heat to painful joints and muscles and to assist the healing process.

Cold therapy: cold can be as soothing as warmth to an inflamed joint, so ice packs are used to relieve pain, increase the circulation, and speed up healing.

Physiotherapists make and fit *splints* for joints which require absolute rest to reduce inflammation.

Physiotherapists help patients who have problems with *walking* as a result of painful joints in the legs and feet, recommending suitable walking aids and footwear.

Physiotherapists teach *relaxation* techniques to help reduce stress and relieve tension, and thus relieve pain.

Many physiotherapists now train in *acupuncture*, and some physiotherapy departments are offering this natural method of treatment to suitable patients.

Occupational therapy and arthritis

Occupational therapists work both in hospitals and in the community, attached to social services departments. They have a wide knowledge of all the gadgets, equipment and adaptations that are available to assist disabled people to live an independent life. They are trained to assess the patient's degree of disability, to recommend aids and adaptations, and to teach patients to use these aids and to find easier ways of performing everyday tasks.

In addition to this very practical work, occupational therapists can educate patients in how to protect their joints and manage their pain, and provide counselling in coming to terms with their disease.

Surgery

If drugs and physical therapy cannot halt the progress of arthritis, and joints become so stiff, painful and deformed that they are virtually useless, and the sufferer's life is adversely affected in all its aspects – social, professional, and domestic – surgery should be considered. One of the most successful surgical advances in the past thirty years has been the replacement of diseased joints with artificial ones, but there are other surgical procedures which may also benefit patients with rheumatic disease.

Arthroplasty (joint replacement)

Artificial joint replacement is indeed one of the surgical success stories of the century. The first hip-joint was replaced in 1938, and since then the procedure and the materials used have been developed and refined until hip-joint replacement has become almost commonplace. Every year 300,000 hip-joints are replaced throughout the world, about 40,000 of them in the UK.

The hip being a ball-and-socket joint, both the worn head of the femur and the socket in the pelvis have to be removed and replaced in a total hip replacement operation. The materials the artificial joints are made of vary according to the preference of the surgeon, but they may be of metal or of high-density plastic, and they are usually cemented into place. There should be immediate relief of pain, and range of movement of the joint should be at least adequate.

Case history

Mr Jenkins, aged sixty-six, suffered badly from osteoarthritis in both hips. In his youth he had been a keen cyclist, and his hip-joints suffered from excessive wear and tear as a result. He eventually became so crippled with pain and stiffness that his family doctor referred him to an orthopaedic surgeon for possible joint replacements.

His X-rays showed extensive damage to both hips, and the surgeon accepted him for replacement, but said he would only do one joint at a time, so that he could observe how Mr Jenkins responded to this type of surgery. Fortunately the waiting list was not long and Mr Jenkins went into hospital after only three months.

After the operation he woke to find himself lying on his back with tubes draining the wound in his hip, and a wedge-shaped pillow between his legs to keep them in the right position. After two days he was helped out of bed by the physiotherapist and shown how to walk again using a walking frame and then two sticks. His hip felt perfectly normal but free of pain, which seemed like a miracle.

After ten days in hospital his stitches were taken out and he was told he could go home in about a week. He managed well at home, walking with a stick, and found he could also manage stairs quite easily. When he returned to hospital for a check-up the surgeon was so pleased with his progress he said he would replace the other hip as soon as he was really fit again.

Knee-joint replacement is now equally successful, 14,000 such operations being done every year in the UK. Being a hinge joint, the ends of the bones have to be re-surfaced, and this is done with metallic plates, with a plastic insert between them to replace the meniscus.

Synovectomy

In rheumatoid and other forms of inflammatory arthritis, the synovial membrane surrounding the joint becomes inflamed. This tissue can be surgically removed in an operation called 'synovectomy'. The pain and swelling will be much reduced, and the synovial membrane will grow again, though in a different form. This operation is sometimes done in rheumatoid arthritis.

Debridement

If small pieces of bone and other loose debris are causing trouble within a joint, they can be removed by a procedure called 'debridement'. This is done with an arthroscope, a small fibre-optic tube through which, when it is inserted into the joint, the surgeon can see to remove any debris. This procedure is sometimes known as 'keyhole surgery'.

Osteotomy

The destruction of bone in arthritis may change the angle at which one bone meets another. This frequently happens in arthritis of the knee-joint, and may also happen in the hip. This can be treated by taking a small piece out of one bone and resetting it so that it meets the other bone at the correct angle.

Arthrodesis

It may not be practicable to replace deformed or unstable joints in younger people, because an artificial joint has a lifespan of only twenty years at most, and a second replacement will last only ten years. It may be necessary to fuse the two bone ends together to correct a deformity and relieve pain, but the joint will be permanently stiff. This fusion of a joint is known as 'arthrodesis'.

Reconstructive surgery

In rheumatic conditions affecting soft tissue, such as tendons, deformities like 'dropped finger' can result from rupture of the tendons. This type of deformity can be corrected surgically by reconstruction of the damaged tendons.

Decompression surgery

Carpal tunnel syndrome is a rheumatic condition in which the sheath covering the tendons of the wrist becomes inflamed and presses on the nerve, making the hand, wrist and arm very painful, particularly at night. The pain can be relieved and the hand and wrist restored to normal function by decompression to relieve the pressure on the trapped median nerve.

Case history

Mr Thompson, a builder aged forty-three, consulted his doctor about a very painful wrist and arm, and numbness and tingling in his fingers. The pain sometimes ran right up his shoulder and kept him awake at night, and he was finding it difficult to work.

His doctor referred him to a rheumatologist, who diagnosed carpal tunnel syndrome and injected his wrist with a cortico-steroid drug to reduce the inflammation. When this did not work, the rheumatologist decided an operation was necessary to free the trapped nerve. This was done under local anaesthetic, and in a couple of months' time Mr Thompson was able to use his hand again freely enough to go back to work.

Success rates for surgery

Surgery is by no means a 'gentle' method of treatment, but in replacement of joints diseased by arthritis its success rate is very high. There is a 1 to 2 per cent risk of infection occurring round the artificial joint which may be due to bacteria already in the patient's body. This can usually be treated effectively with antibiotics.

There is also the slight risk of a pulmonary embolism – formation of a blood clot in the leg or pelvis which travels to the lung. This is a risk in most operations, and doctors are accustomed to dealing with it.

The great boon to patients of joint replacement surgery is the relief of pain which has seemed interminable and intolerable, and the ability to use the joint again almost normally. This type of surgery is continually developing and genuinely offers a new lease of life to people suffering from arthritis.

CHAPTER 7

The natural therapies and arthritis

Introducing the 'gentle alternatives'

Since the conventional drugs prescribed to control the pain and inflammation of moderate-to-severe arthritis have such unpleasant – not to say dangerous – side-effects, it is hardly surprising that sufferers are anxious to find gentler, safer methods of controlling their symptoms, and turn with a degree of hope to the so-called 'natural', or complementary, therapies. And as medical science has so far failed to identify the cause of inflammatory arthritis – although a number of theories are being tested by research – sufferers are bound to ask themselves if practitioners of the alternative natural therapies have succeeded where conventional medicine has failed in finding both cause and cure.

For a long time the medical profession was antagonistic towards the natural therapies, but now more and more doctors are becoming interested in their possibilities, and some have trained in certain natural treatments, such as homoeopathy and acupuncture. If you are thinking of 'going natural', so to speak, and if your family doctor is already treating your arthritis by conventional methods, you should consult your doctor first, and discuss the natural therapies which are most suitable for you.

Even if your doctor has reservations about alternative medicine, and you decide to go ahead anyway, you should keep him or her informed in case the drugs being prescribed for you are likely to interact with any natural remedy you may take. You should also tell your natural therapist which conventional drugs you are taking.

What is natural therapy?

The natural methods of treating disease are all based on the following principles.

- The body has a natural ability to heal and regulate itself.
- A human being is not simply a machine, like a car, but a subtle and complex blend of body, mind and emotions, and any or all of these factors may play a part in health problems. In other words, each individual is not a random collection of parts, but a fully integrated 'whole'. The term 'holistic medicine' is based on this concept, and implies treating each patient as a whole being whose intellect and emotions, or spirit, are as important to health as the body.
- Environmental and social conditions are just as important as a person's physical and psychological make-up, and may have just as much impact on his or her health.
- Treating the root cause or causes of a problem is more important than treating the obvious immediate symptoms. Merely treating symptoms may cover up the underlying problem and make it worse, so that it occurs again later in a more serious form.
- Every individual is unique, and cannot be treated in the same way as everyone else.
- Healing is quicker and more effective if people take central responsibility for their own health, and are

actively involved in the healing process. (A good therapist will, however, recognize when a patient needs to let go and place this responsibility in the hands of someone else.)

- Good health is a state of emotional, mental, spiritual and physical balance. Balance is fundamental to the concept of health in natural therapy: ill-health results from a state of imbalance, or 'dis-ease'. The Chinese describe this concept of balance as the principle of *yin* and *yang*.

- There is a natural healing force in the universe. In the West this is known by the Latin phrase *vis medicatrix naturae* (healing power of nature), in China as *qi* or *chi*, in Japan as *ki*, and in India as *prana*. Anyone can draw on this healing force, and it is a natural therapist's skill to activate it in the patient, or help patients to activate it in themselves.

The essence of all natural therapies is the same, and follows closely the principles of medicine as it was practised in ancient Greece and Egypt: that the best approach is the one that is softest and most gentle, that avoids dangerous and invasive procedures, that treats the patient as a whole person, and encourages patients to take an active part in their own recovery and to maintain their health.

The aims and principles of natural therapy are not so far removed from those of conventional medicine, which also recognizes the close links between the mind and the body – the *psyche* and the *soma* – in health and disease. It seems only logical that the skills and knowledge of practitioners in both disciplines should be regarded as complementary to each other, and that they should be encouraged to co-operate, to the ultimate benefit of patients.

What natural therapies are there?

The wide range of natural methods of healing can be divided into two broad categories: the physical therapies that treat the body, and the psychological therapies that treat the mind and emotions. Some therapies, of course, fall into both categories. Those that are helpful in arthritis are listed in alphabetical order in the box below. Some are therapies you can practise yourself after some initial instruction. Others should only be applied by a trained practitioner.

Sufferers from arthritis need treatment that will relieve pain and reduce inflammation, and also relieve the stress that can provoke an attack. This is particularly true of rheumatoid arthritis, which is an inflammatory disease of the joints that is sometimes triggered by stress. But it is also true of osteoarthritis in its advanced stage when the tissue around the joint becomes inflamed by the outgrowths of bone in the joint.

Pain is also likely to be severe and debilitating at this stage, causing stress. Thus any method of treatment that will effectively control pain will also reduce stress. Equally, treatment that encourages relaxation and relief of tension will enable the patient to tolerate pain more easily. This is why some dentists play soothing music to tense patients with a low pain threshold.

The natural therapies that will probably benefit sufferers from arthritis are: acupuncture; moxibustion and acupressure, which operate on the same principle as acupuncture; naturopathy; dietary manipulation; homoeopathy; herbal medicine; aromatherapy; reflexology; yoga and t'ai chi; autogenics; relaxation; hypnotherapy; biofeedback; and meditation. These therapies will be discussed in the next two chapters.

While osteopathy, chiropractic and other manipulative therapies such as massage and Alexander technique also claim to benefit arthritics they should be viewed with great caution, as manipulating or massaging an inflamed and painful joint wrongly can do more harm than good. This is why it is so important to seek advice from your doctor before embarking on a course of natural therapy.

Some of these natural therapies may also be effective in treating various rheumatic conditions. Fibromyalgia and bursitis have both been reported to respond well to acupuncture, for example. But, again, you would be wise to consult your own doctor first.

The natural therapies and arthritis	
Physical therapies	**Psychological therapies**
Acupuncture	Autogenics
Acupressure	Biofeedback
Aromatherapy	Hypnotherapy
Dietary manipulation	Meditation
Herbal medicine	Relaxation therapy
Homoeopathy	
Moxibustion	
Naturopathy	
Reflexology	
T'ai chi	
Yoga	

CHAPTER 8

Treating your body

Physical therapies for arthritis

Of the various natural physical therapies that are claimed to be successful in treating arthritis, three have been proved by scientific research to be of some benefit. They are:

- Acupuncture
- Homoeopathy
- Dietary or nutritional therapy

Acupuncture

Acupuncture, and its 'spin-off' moxibustion, are traditional Chinese therapies, their use having been recorded as long ago as 475–221BC in an ancient medical treatise *Nei Jing (The Canon of Medicine)*. This treatise states: 'Moxibustion may be applied when and where acupuncture alone proves ineffective'.

Chinese traditional medicine is based on the belief that there is a life force, or force of nature, called *chi* energy, and that this controls the main organs and systems of the body. This energy moves from one organ to another, always along the same route or pathways, called 'meridians'. There are fourteen meridians, each with acupuncture points which are the entrances and exits for the vital energy that circulates in the meridians. An acupuncturist has to know not only the relevant meridians to which the acupuncture points belong but also the exact anatomical sites of the acupuncture points.

After diagnosis of the patient's condition, treatment is given by inserting needles into the acupuncture points of the meridian leading to the affected organ. These points may be some distance away: for example, the meridian leading to the large intestine starts in the fingertips, and that leading to the spleen originates in the big toe. There may be as many as sixty-seven acupuncture points on one meridian.

According to a manual produced by the Chinese Traditional Medical College and Research Institute of Shanghai there are 361 *jing* points along the fourteen meridians, as well as fifty-eight *qi* or extraordinary points, not yet classified. Great emphasis has evidently always been placed on accurate selection of the points. An eminent Chinese practitioner of the thirteenth century once remarked: 'It is necessary to consider five points in order to select one properly'.

The needles used nowadays are made of stainless steel or gold, but the earliest acupuncture needles used in China were made of stone, bone and bamboo. A variety of bronze articles, including needles, from the Shang and Chouh dynasties (16th–8th centuries BC) have been discovered, and four gold and five silver needles were found in 1968 in the tomb of Prince Ching of Chungsan, dating back to the 2nd century BC. There were originally nine types of needle, each serving a different purpose, including one large needle specifically for treating painful joints.

While the traditional objective of acupuncture is to treat the underlying cause of the disease, it has been developed in recent years mainly as an analgesic and anaesthetic procedure. It is now used routinely in Chinese hospitals as an anaesthetic for surgery, sometimes combined with herbs or with Western drugs,

Case history

Mr Wilson, aged fifty-seven, had suffered from recurring attacks of rheumatoid arthritis for about four years. The knee-joint in his right leg was always badly affected, and continued to be painful after the acute flare-up had passed off. The anti-inflammatory drugs he was taking didn't help much, and when his family doctor tried him on a more powerful 'second-line' drug, he found the side-effects so unpleasant he refused to take it, although the pain in his knee was making walking difficult and disturbing his sleep.

Mr Wilson's doctor decided to refer him to the consultant rheumatologist at the local hospital, who suggested he attend the pain clinic there. To his surprise, Mr Wilson was seen by an acupuncturist, who explained that he could treat his pain by inserting slender steel needles in his leg, near the knee-joint, and manipulating them. He would need treatment once a week for about two months.

Although he was sceptical Mr Wilson returned the following week for his first session. Unexpectedly, he hardly felt the needles being inserted, though he had a sensation of numbness in his leg. The acupuncturist told him the pain would go for only a brief period at first, but he would be pain free for longer periods after each session, and eventually his knee should be normal. Also there would be no side-effects after treatment.

In six weeks Mr Wilson's knee was much less painful, and after two months he reported the pain had gone altogether.

and frequently in Western hospitals and pain clinics to control intractable pain.

No one – not even the Chinese – is quite sure how it works, but one theory is that when the needles are inserted into the acupuncture points and manipulated they release into the bloodstream chemicals called *endorphins*, which act in the same way as the strong painkilling drug morphine. Another theory is that the stimulation by needles blocks the nerve pathways that carry pain messages to the brain.

Moxibustion is the application of heat from slowly burning *moxa*-wool sticks held near the diseased area or an acupuncture point. Moxa cones can also be placed directly on or above the area. Moxa-wool is made from the shredded dried leaves of the Chinese wormwood plant.

Acupressure is a combination of massage and acupuncture, given with strong fingertip movements over the acupuncture points. It is believed by some to be the precursor of acupuncture.

Acupuncture will relieve the pain of inflamed joints and muscles, but it will not cure arthritis or restore the damage caused to bones by the disease process. However, if given by properly qualified practitioners – and they now include many doctors – it can bring great relief from pain and stress.

Homoeopathy

Like acupuncture, homoeopathy has acquired a measure of respectability with the medical profession, and in Britain is available free on the National Health Service. There are five homoeopathic hospitals in the UK, and around a thousand doctors regularly practise homoeopathy. In spite of a number of research studies that have proved it to be an effective method of treatment, medical opinion still differs. Some doctors believe, that its value lies in the so-called 'placebo effect'. That is, patients will respond to a neutral substance – a placebo – if they believe strongly enough in its power to do them good. But more doctors are now seeing this as a positive factor, and probable evidence of the power of the mind to influence the body.

Case history

The late Dr Margery Blackie, one of the great teachers of homoeopathy and physician to the Queen from 1968 until her death in 1981, described in *Classical Homoeopathy* the case of a sixty-three year old woman who, when she first saw her, was in constant pain, getting upstairs only with extreme difficulty and able to walk very little, even on the level.

Her rheumatic condition had started when she was sixteen, and had got much worse after she suffered a perforated appendix at twenty-eight. In spite of every kind of conventional medical treatment the disease had progressed.

With continuous homoeopathic treatment her pain became much less, she often had pain-free spells, and she was able to walk and to climb stairs quite easily.

Homoeopathy (meaning 'like disease') is based on the principle of 'treating like with like'. This 'law of similars' was developed by a German doctor, Samuel Hahnemann, in the early nineteenth century, after he noticed that a herbal remedy from the bark of the *Cinchona* tree actually produced the symptoms of malaria – the disease it was intended to cure. He deduced that a substance that produced symptoms of a certain illness could be used to treat that illness, and his view was underpinned by the discovery that Cinchona tree bark contains *quinine*, which is indeed used to treat malaria.

Hahnemann believed homoeopathic remedies should be given in very small doses, and experimented on himself and his family for many years using a wide range of natural substances in very dilute forms. He believed in treating the whole person – mind and spirit as well as body – so his approach was holistic.

Homoeopaths today still follow this approach, interviewing patients exhaustively before tailoring a course of treatment to their individual requirements. Their aim is to encourage the healing force within people to restore the balance that has been disturbed, producing symptoms of disease.

The remedies they prescribe are very dilute preparations of natural substances – obtained from animals, plants and minerals – which would produce symptoms of the disease to be treated. The process of dilution is effected by vigorous shaking, or 'succussion', which homoeopaths believe produces changes in the water molecules which enable them to 'memorize' the substance being diluted. Conventional medical practitioners are generally sceptical about this theory despite recent research in France and elsewhere which has appeared to show this to be so.

There are a number of homoeopathic remedies effective for arthritis and rheumatism, including *Argentum nitricum*, *aurum metallicum* (homoeopathic gold), *causticum*, and *Rhus tox*. None of these has side-effects, unlike many of the drugs used to treat arthritis.

Homoeopathic remedies can be bought off the shelf in health food stores and pharmacies but in the UK the watchdog organization the Consumers' Association advised readers of their magazine *Which? Way to Health* in 1992 that shop assistants may not be adequately trained to give advice about suitable remedies, the leaflets accompanying the products sold are not clear enough, and may even be missing, and there is often inadequate information on product packs.

Qualified homoeopaths spend a great deal of time questioning and observing their patients in order to get an overall picture of their personalities as well as their complaints before planning a course of treatment unique to each individual's needs. Consulting a homoeopath personally rather than buying a homoeopathic remedy over-the-counter, however well-intentioned and well-informed the sales staff may be, is therefore more likely to be effective.

Dietary therapy

It is generally recognized that diet has a role to play in the treatment of arthritis, if only to reduce weight and thus relieve the burden painful weight-bearing joints have to carry.

A great deal of research has been going on all over the world during the past few decades into the value of food supplements in rheumatoid arthritis, and into the possibility that certain foods may provoke or exacerbate the symptoms of rheumatoid arthritis because sufferers are sensitive to them, or intolerant of them.

Rheumatoid arthritis has been specifically the subject of this research, being the most common form of inflammatory arthritis. Osteoarthritis, being degenerative, seldom benefits from attempts to reduce inflammation by dietary manipulation unless it is in its advanced stage. Sufferers do benefit from a weight-reducing diet, however.

Food supplements

Scientific research has shown that fish oil and evening primrose oil are the supplements most likely to help reduce inflammation in rheumatoid arthritis.

The best sources of fish oil are oily fish such as salmon, herring and mackerel; white fish like cod, haddock and plaice contain less oil. You would need to eat 8 ounces (250 grams) of oily fish or 20 ounces (600 grams) of white fish every day to get enough benefit, so a fish oil supplement is a much more practicable alternative. You need to take a daily dose of fish oil for up to six months for it to be effective, and if you find it eases your symptoms you must continue taking it regularly, as the benefit will cease if you stop.

Evening primrose oil has been proved to have anti-inflammatory effects, and must also be taken for three to six months to be of real benefit. There is no point in taking it *as well as* fish oil though. This will only increase your calorie intake and help you put on weight.

Research has also been done into the possible benefits of other popular food supplements for arthritis. While honey, garlic and vitamins are good in themselves they have no proven benefit in rheumatoid arthritis. Kelp, royal jelly, ginseng, and cider vinegar – good for other things – are also of no proven value for arthritis. And while extract of New Zealand green-lipped mussel has been popular with some patients research studies have not revealed any improvement as a result of taking it either.

Food intolerance

Many research studies have shown that the symptoms of rheumatoid arthritis have been aggravated by particular foods, and some researchers believe that it is caused by an intolerance to certain foods. Those most commonly implicated are milk and dairy products, wheat, gluten, corn, beef, coffee, citrus fruits, tomatoes and peanuts.

To find out what foods may be responsible, the patient is put on what is called an 'elimination diet' – one which will identify the culprits by a process of elimination. This may be quite a lengthy business, taking up to six months.

First the patient will be given a very basic diet, which may vary according to the practitioner's methods but which will probably include so-called 'neutral' foods like lamb, rice, cabbage, carrots, pears and filtered water. If the symptoms improve greatly after two weeks on this diet, other foods are introduced in a carefully planned sequence to see which ones may make the symptoms return. Once these have been discovered, they are excluded from the patient's diet.

General diet for rheumatoid arthritis
The most healthy diet for anyone suffering from rheumatoid arthritis is one that is low in total fat (but includes some polyunsaturated fat), low in sugar, low in salt, low in alcohol and high in fibre.

This is the diet recommended for general health: cutting out sweet things like biscuits, cakes, pastries, and puddings, cutting down on red meat and meat products, milk and dairy products, butter and eggs, avoiding fried foods but eating plenty of fish, fresh fruit and vegetables, wholemeal bread, wholegrain cereals, pasta and rice.

Small amounts of polyunsaturated fats like margarine and peanut butter can be included, as well as low-fat cheese, skimmed milk, low-fat yoghurt and fromage frais, and protein from chicken, pulses and nuts.

Diet as self-help
The great advantage of a dietary regime in rheumatoid arthritis is that the sufferer, after seeking advice from an expert practitioner, can take control of his or her own treatment. It is important that an elimination diet should only be undertaken under the supervision of a doctor, dietitian, or other qualified professional, as nutrition must be carefully maintained – especially so in the case of children so that their development is not impeded.

Practitioners

Many doctors are specializing in the effects of diet and of other environmental factors on various diseases, and rheumatologists have an interest in the role of diet in inflammatory arthritis. Some dietitians also specialize in this branch of healthcare.

Naturopathy is said to be very effective in the treatment of arthritis. Like other natural therapies, it treats the whole person, aims to identify the cause underlying the symptoms, and encourages the body to use its own healing force. According to this therapy, food should be eaten in its natural state so far as possible.

Other physical therapies

Herbal medicine, reflexology, yoga, t'ai chi, and aromatherapy are all natural therapies that are worth considering, although they have not been subjected to extensive scientific research.

Herbal medicine

Treatment with plants or plant extracts is an ancient skill, still actively practised in many countries, particularly China, and arthritis is one of the many diseases it claims to benefit. A remedy called *Devil's claw* is said to be very effective, for example.

Some remedies are given product licences by the controlling authorities in different countries (The Medicines Control Agency in Britain) to be sold as medicines. Others are sold as foods, and are covered by the food laws (the Food Safety Act in the UK). The risk you take in buying a herbal remedy over the counter is that it may not suit you or it may interact with a drug you are taking, so it is really essential to consult a qualified herbalist who will examine you carefully and prescribe for you individually.

If you do buy a herbal remedy over the counter in Britain look to see if the letters 'PL' (product licence) are on the container, as this at least means its qualities have been assessed and approved. More research into herbal remedies is needed to ensure that all those sold over the counter are safe.

Reflexology

This is another ancient skill, possibly originating in China, and based on roughly the same principles as acupuncture. It is a form of massage of areas of the feet, each area having a specific link with other parts of the body – either through meridians or other 'energy' lines (opinions differ). Thus massaging the big toe can relieve headache. No trials of reflexology have been held, so there is no scientific proof of its efficacy, but doctors believe it can do no harm, and may certainly do some good. A modern 'high-tech' version gaining popularity is Vacuflex which uses a vacuum pump and suction pads to achieve its effect.

Yoga and t'ai chi

These are both forms of gentle controlled exercise that can benefit arthritis by keeping stiff joints mobile, and by encouraging relaxation and countering stress.

Yoga is widely practised throughout the Western world, and classes taken by trained instructors are not hard to find. The great violinist Yehudi Menuhin took up yoga when his playing was threatened by a rheumatic condition called 'frozen shoulder'. His shoulder was freed, and he says yoga helped his playing enormously.

In Britain the Yoga Biomedical Trust is carrying out a number of research projects at special clinics set up at the Royal Homoeopathic Hospital in London to investigate such benefits.

T'ai chi is another ancient Chinese art which you can see being practised – usually first thing in the morning –

in the streets of most towns and cities in China. It has been well described as 'meditation in motion'. It consists of a series of slow, dance-like movements which are intended to make people focus on their minds and emotions as well as their bodies. It too is widely taught and practised in the West.

Aromatherapy

This treatment uses the highly scented oils which give the plants from which they are extracted their individual smells. These are plant essences, or 'essential oils'. This, too, is an ancient art which has been revived this century and has become increasingly popular. Many nurses have trained in this therapy and it is provided in many hospitals, where its benefits for a wide range of illnesses are becoming increasingly recognized.

Treatment may be in the form of massage, compresses, baths and inhalations. Aromatherapists claim that their treatment can benefit almost any disease, including arthritis and rheumatism, as well as nervous and emotional problems such as stress and depression. There are virtually no side-effects, and all age groups – particularly the elderly – can benefit. It can also be used in the home on a self-help basis.

A word of warning: never eat or drink essential oils, and don't use them undiluted. Some oils are dangerous for pregnant women and children so read instructions carefully or, better still, consult a qualified aromatherapist.

Until recently, little research had been done on aromatherapy, but now studies into the reasons for its obvious effectiveness are being carried out all over the world.

CHAPTER 9

Treating your mind and emotions

Psychological therapies for arthritis

A diagnosis of rheumatoid arthritis or osteoarthritis can amount to a sentence of chronic pain. In a report entitled *Arthritis: The Painful Challenge*, published by the UK organization Arthritis Care in 1989, a patient is quoted as saying: 'You are never on your own . . . You always have your pain for company.' Chronic pain causes great stress if it cannot be controlled, and a vicious circle is created by the fact that stress can act as a trigger for acute attacks of rheumatoid arthritis.

The aim of natural psychological therapies in arthritis must therefore be to reduce the stress caused by pain, as this will also reduce the pain, and to reduce any stress that may trigger flare-ups of inflammatory arthritis. The natural therapies that can help to break the vicious circle of pain and stress are autogenics, relaxation techniques, hypnotherapy and biofeedback. Meditation may also be beneficial.

Autogenics

The word 'autogenic' means originating from within the individual, and in the context of natural therapy it means exercising the mind in order to restore the health of the body. There are similarities with yoga and meditation.

Autogenic therapy is based on six simple mental exercises whose purpose is to relieve stress and encourage the healing process. Three main positions must be adopted so that the exercises can be done in familiar situations – for example at work, in the train, or while lying down. They are the simple sitting position, the armchair position, and the reclining position.

The six mental exercises concentrate on heaviness (thinking a limb feels heavy), warmth, the heartbeat, breathing, warmth in the stomach, and coolness of the forehead. A therapist will first teach them in groups, asking patients to practise the exercises at home, so that eventually they will be able to do them whenever it is convenient.

Autogenic therapy originated in Germany in the late 1920s, developed by a Dr Johannes Schulz in Berlin who used hypnotism to treat his patients. Observing how much they benefited from hypnotic relaxation, he devised a series of mental exercises that would produce the same effects. They proved so successful that the system spread to the rest of Europe, North America, and Japan. It was introduced into the UK in the 1970s.

Relaxation therapy

You have read in Chapter 4 that learning to relax is one good way to help yourself cope with stress. All you need is twenty minutes of peace and quiet, preferably in a room by yourself, where you can lie flat on the floor.

The technique is to empty your mind of all negative thoughts, to visualize the beauties of a tranquil scene, and to imagine the sounds of nature that epitomize that scene and bring it to life in your mind.

Having set your scene to create peace and tranquillity of mind, next begin to relax all your muscles, taking one group at a time. Start with your toes and feet and continue with your fingers and hands, first contracting and then relaxing a muscle group so that eventually all your limbs feel heavy and inert. If someone lifted one of your arms it would just flop back on to the floor.

Continue the process of contracting and relaxing muscle groups all the way up the body, even to your eyebrows and forehead, and when you are completely relaxed just lie there for a while as if letting your body sink through the floor. Then bring yourself back to reality slowly and gently, without any hurry.

You can combine the relaxation with breathing exercises which will also help you to overcome any tensions. When you are under stress, your breathing is usually quick and shallow, from the upper chest only, which means that you don't take enough air into your lungs or expel the waste products out of the lungs properly. You need to learn to breathe from the diaphragm – like actors and singers – so that you expand your lungs to their full extent and take in sufficient air to feed the heart with the oxygen it needs to beat strongly.

The diaphragm is a strong band of muscle separating the cavities of the chest and stomach. You can feel it with your hand expanding and contracting as you breathe. You have to learn to control it so that when you breathe in air enters to the very bottom of your lungs, and you can feel the foot of your rib cage expanding. Equally, when you breathe out you contract the diaphragm so that it expels as much air as possible from your lungs and gets rid of all the waste products.

You should practise controlling your diaphragmatic breathing until you can breathe in to a count of three, hold your breath for a count of three, breathe out to a count of three, and hold it for another count of three. Keep your shoulder muscles relaxed – don't let them hunch up and feel tense.

If you need any help with these exercises you should

consult a physical therapist. Once you have mastered both relaxation techniques and breathing exercises you will be amazed at how much calmer and more in control of yourself you feel. You will also find that your pain is not so bad.

Hypnotherapy

'Hypnosis has been with us a long time, but hypnotherapists are still battling for respect', an article in the UK Consumers' Association magazine *Which? Way to Health* declared in December 1993. It went on to say that research – and hypnotherapy is the most researched of all the natural therapies – has failed to prove that being in a hypnotic trance is any different from deep relaxation, meditation or being lost in a book.

In hypnosis you are fully conscious but deeply relaxed, with your mind focused. A patient in a state of trance becomes suggestible – the hypnotherapist can help to solve problems by suggesting possible solutions to them, as well as changes in the patient's behaviour. Any suggestions made by the hypnotherapist during hypnosis can be agreed on beforehand. It is said that most patients remember everything after waking up from hypnosis and, as with all the natural therapies, the aim is to help you to help yourself.

Hypnosis is used not only to treat psychological problems like fears and phobias, but also to relieve pain and stress, and to treat addictions and eating disorders, as well as certain skin conditions. Many doctors and psychologists use hypnosis as part of a whole treatment programme.

As there is no law, in Britain at least, to prevent people calling themselves hypnotherapists, whether they are trained or not, it is wise to make sure that you consult one who is genuine. The next chapter explains in detail how to set about finding any natural therapist who is properly trained and qualified.

It has been proved that hypnotherapy can relieve pain, and also remove it altogether in a patient who is put into a deep trance.

Biofeedback

This should more accurately be called 'biofeedback training', because it is a method of teaching someone how to control the involuntary responses of the body – such as the raising and lowering of blood pressure and of body temperature – which happen as an automatic response to excessive heat and cold, or to emotions such as fear, anger, hate, anxiety and depression.

The therapist measures the patient's involuntary responses with various pieces of electrical equipment, such as a hand-held thermometer which can show the presence of headache or migraine from the temperature of the hand, or an electric skin resistance gauge (similar to a lie detector) which reacts to the sweat of fear or anxiety on the skin.

The measurements are made known to the patient by a system of lights or sound. The therapist then teaches the patient how to control his or her automatic reactions, using the lighting or sound signals on the machine as a guide to the degree of success.

Biofeedback is a prime example of using the power of the mind over the body to restore it to health. It is very popular in the USA, where it has been extensively used and studied by psychologists, and it has also been used in the UK to treat addictions to smoking, eating and drinking, to cure stammering, and to treat migraine. If it can be used to control stress successfully, it should be effective in treating all stress-related diseases, including rheumatoid arthritis.

Meditation

Meditation has been practised in India and much of Asia for thousands of years, and yoga is an offshoot of this method of finding a still, calm centre in the storms of life. It is believed to be the best method of self-help, in that people practising meditation do it by concentrating their thoughts and controlling their body until both mind and body are in a state of peace and harmony.

The method is similar to the relaxation techniques and breathing exercises already described, and the objective is much the same – to clear the mind of troublesome thoughts and fill it with one calm and beautiful thought or idea.

If stress is a problem for you, this is another way of dealing with it that is worth considering. Classes are widely available in the UK, usually at adult education centres.

Pain and the mind

Perhaps the most distressing feature of arthritis is the pain it causes – both acute pain in the active phases of the disease, and persistent long-term pain which the sufferer has to learn to live with. Pain is both physically and emotionally exhausting, and because of that it can cause deep depression. Powerful pain-killing drugs usually have unpleasant side-effects, so it is all the more essential to try and find more natural and gentle ways of controlling pain.

Everyone feels pain differently. Some people can tolerate pain easily, while others get very upset by the pain of a minor injury. This is known as 'pain tolerance'.

The 'pain threshold' is the moment when you first feel pain, and this is usually much the same in everyone. But the fact that the ability to tolerate pain varies so much from one person to another suggests that mental attitude may have something to do with it.

It is well known, for example, that soldiers severely wounded in battle often don't feel pain until after the action is over and they have time to think about their injuries. This is an illustration of the fact that you feel pain less if your attention is distracted by something more urgent and important.

As mentioned earlier, it is also known that a 'placebo' – an innocuous substance, like chalk – given in place of a painkilling drug without the patient's knowledge, can relieve the pain because the patient believes it is a painkiller. This so-called 'placebo effect' is another example of the power of mind over matter.

The patient's anxiety about his or her pain and illness can be relieved by a placebo given by an encouraging doctor, which demonstrates that pain and mood are closely linked, and a positive attitude on the part of both patient and doctor can help to overcome pain.

Self-help in controlling pain

There are a number of ways in which one can make a conscious mental effort to control one's pain, as described below.

Operant conditioning

People in great pain attract a good deal of sympathy and attention, which they unconsciously enjoy and regard as a reward for their suffering. Eventually they may use their pain to gain specific rewards, and this is known by specialists in human behaviour as an 'operant': something you use to manipulate people for your own ends.

The process can, however, be 'conditioned' – or stopped – by using the same technique but in reverse. In other words, people who use pain to demand attention and 'rewards' beyond their needs must be ignored until the demands stop and behaviour becomes normal again. This sounds hard-hearted, but it is how 'operant conditioning' works – a case of being cruel to be kind.

If you recognize that you are using your own pain to obtain rewards, you can condition yourself by making a conscious effort to change this behaviour, perhaps by being more considerate of the people around you, or by immersing yourself in a hobby you enjoy, or by voluntary or fund-raising work for a charity that supports people with your disease. By active effort to take your attention off your pain and to focus it elsewhere, you will be able to tolerate your pain better.

Healing imagery
This is a self-help method developed in the United States by Dr Martin L. Rossman, practising in California. Patients with arthritis are advised first to use relaxation techniques to reduce stress and muscle tension, then to create an image in their minds of their disease, focusing first on one affected joint and comparing it with others, then visualizing the diseased joint as normal.

If the arthritis is widespread, the patient can visualize the disease process as it affects the whole body, and imagine healing taking place. Patients are asked to practise deep relaxation and healing imagery for ten to fifteen minutes at least twice a day for a period of three weeks, and then to assess their progress.

Dr Rossman lays emphasis on the importance of a healthy lifestyle, and on vividly imagining yourself to be 'healthy, flexible, recovered, and leading a life you can enjoy'. He quotes the case history of a man with a very painful, inflamed wrist who first visualized his wrist bones as having sharp, jagged edges which grated on each other as they moved, and then contrasted this image with one of rounded wrist bones with soft pads between them that allowed his wrist to move smoothly and painlessly. By practising this healing imagery regularly, he was able to reduce his discomfort greatly while his wrist healed.

Self-efficacy

This term was used at Stanford Arthritis Center in America to describe the sense of control over their circumstances that people suffering from arthritis need to develop. The sense of helplessness and depression that often accompany persistent pain can actually make that pain worse, so patients on a self-management course were taught to play a positive role in their treatment programme by participating in decisions taken about their care, designing their own exercise regimes, and evaluating the various methods of treatment provided. This active role gave them a feeling of control over their circumstances and a belief in their own 'self-efficacy', or ability to take control of their health.

Those completing this course apparently had less pain and depression and joints that were more mobile than before, and even after twenty months suffered less pain and consulted their doctors less frequently. A theory for the positive results of self-efficacy has been put forward by a Stanford psychologist, Albert Bandura, who claims that when people feel they have gained control over a stressful situation, their bodies release lower levels of *catecholamines* – chemicals produced in response to stress which may increase physical discomfort.

Information and advice

If you are interested in any of these and other newly developed psychological methods of controlling your own pain, your doctor should be able to put you in touch with a psychologist or psychotherapist who specializes in natural methods of pain control, and who could teach you to help yourself. The consultant in charge of the pain clinic at your local hospital should also be able to give you more information and advice.

Managing your own pain

If you have persistent pain that you have to learn to live with, it is vital to try and keep it under control so that it doesn't rule your life. The power of the mind over the body is something you can learn to understand and to use.

Always remember the value of relaxation and deep-breathing techniques in overcoming both physical and mental tension and thus reducing pain. Don't forget that gentle exercise will also relieve stiff and painful joints, and a little gentle massage may help as well.

Applying warmth to a painful part of the body, in the form of a heat pad or a hot-water bottle, is one of the most trusted natural ways of relieving pain, but cold can also help, and ice-cubes in a waterproof bag placed on the affected part can reduce inflammation and pain as well. If heat doesn't work, it is well worth trying cold as an alternative.

If you bang your elbow on a piece of furniture it is instinctive to rub the bruised and painful joint, and it is on this principle that *transcutaneous electrical nerve stimulation* (TENS) has been developed. This form of therapy is given by an electrical apparatus that stimulates the nerve fibres of a painful part by passing an electrical current through the skin into them. Thin 'C' fibres carry pain messages to the brain, but thicker 'A' fibres can pass messages more quickly, and when stimulated can block the slower 'C' fibre pain signals. This is known as the 'gate theory' of pain control.

TENS therapy is frequently used in hospitals, usually given by physiotherapists who are trained in electrotherapy, but the apparatus can be prescribed by family doctors for their patients to buy and use at home. Versions are on open sale in most countries.

All this means that someone in pain does not have to rely on pain-killing drugs, but has the choice of using both physical and psychological natural methods of therapy to manage that pain. And learning that one can have a positive effect on one's own health by exerting the power of mind over matter is perhaps the greatest morale-booster of all.

CHAPTER 10

How to find and choose a natural therapist

Tips and guidelines for finding reliable help

It is unfortunately not as easy as it should be to find the right therapist. Although natural medicine is enjoying a boom and everyone seems to want to use it, diversity, competition between groups and duplication within therapies has made the task a difficult one in most countries where their popularity is on the increase. It is the main purpose of the *Natural Way* series to help you find the right gentle therapy for your condition – but finding the right practitioner or therapist is in some ways the harder task.

The best answer is almost always personal recommendation, and this applies as much to doctors as non-medical practitioners. Go to someone a friend or someone you trust has recommended. As a rule of thumb it cannot be bettered. But if you cannot get a good recommendation, what next? There are several options.

● Go to your local doctor's clinic or health centre and ask their advice. It may take some courage and you may not get a sympathetic response but it is worth a try, and you may get a pleasant surprise: you may find they have the very person you need – either someone who helps at the clinic or to whom patients are referred (which means, in countries with a state health service, possibly free treatment).

- Your nearest natural health centre may be able to help, or you may know of a natural health practitioner who is not the right person for you but who may be prepared to recommend someone else who may be. This way is not as good as personal recommendation but therapists who specialize in natural therapy tend to know who else is at work in their area and, more important, who is any good.

- You can get the names of centres and individual practitioners to approach from health food shops, business telephone directories or local listings in newspapers, magazines, citizen advice and information centres and libraries. Computer networks also have lists.

  A particularly good bet is a natural health centre in your area which has several practitioners with different skills working at it. The better centres have a system where a patient contacting them for help will be offered a consultation in which his or her case is considered by a panel of practitioners and a therapy or therapies and a therapist or therapists recommended. Such an approach is still in its infancy, though, so it may be hard to find.

- Failing a local recommendation or the availability of an enlightened group practice, the next step is to contact any of the national therapy 'umbrella' organizations and ask for their list(s) of registered organizations or practitioners. Their addresses are in Appendix A. They may charge for their lists (especially for postage and packing) and insist you select not only which therapy but also, because there is still no one recognized organization for each therapy in many countries, for which particular organization you want a members' list. If you can afford it, ask for the lot.

Ten ways of finding a therapist

- Word of mouth (usually the best method)
- Your local family medical centres
- Your local natural health centres
- Your local health food shops
- Health farms and beauty treatment centres
- Local patient support groups
- National therapy organizations (but see below)
- Computer networks (you need a 'modem')
- Public libraries and information centres
- Local directories, newspapers and magazines.

Checking professional organizations

It is always a good idea to check on a therapist's professional background, especially if you are picking a name from a list rather than following a recommendation from a friend. However, just because a therapist belongs to an organization doesn't mean he or she comes with a guarantee. Some organizations do no more vetting of their members than making sure they've paid their membership fees.

Before you even choose your therapist therefore you should check the status of the individual associations or professional organizations whose names you have got. A good association will publish the information clearly and simply in the same booklet as its members' list. Few seem to, however, and so you may have to ring them up or write to them. The following are the sort of questions you should try and get answered.

- When was the association founded? (Groups spring up all the time and you may find it useful to know if they have been going fifty years or started yesterday.)

- How many members does it have? (Size will give you a good idea of its public acceptance and genuine aims.)
- Is it a charity or educational trust – with a formal constitution, an elected committee and published accounts – or is it a private limited company? (Private companies can be secretive and self-serving.)
- Is it part of a larger network of professional organizations? (Groups that go their own way are on balance more suspect than those who 'join in'.)
- Does the association have a code of ethics, complaints mechanism and disciplinary procedures? If so, what are they?
- Is the association linked to one particular school or college? (One that is may have no independent assessment of its membership; the head of the association may also be head of the college.)
- What are the criteria for membership? (If it is graduation from one particular school or college the same problem arises as above.)
- Are members covered by professional indemnity insurance against accident and malpractice?

Checking training and qualifications

Next you may want to try and satisfy yourself about the individual therapist's training and qualifications. A good listing will, again, describe the qualifications and say what the initials after every member's name mean. Yet again, few seem to. So it's a case of ringing or writing to find out. Questions to ask are the following:

- How long is the training?
- Is it full or part time?
- Does it include seeing patients under supervision?
- Is the qualification recognized?
- If so, by whom?

The British Medical Association's opinion

In its long-awaited second report into the practice of natural medicine in Britain, published in June 1993, the British Medical Association (BMA) recommended that anyone seeking the help of a non-conventional therapist – doctor or patient – should ask the following questions:

- Is the therapist registered with a professional organization?
- Does the professional organization have
  - a public register?
  - a code of practice?
  - an effective disciplinary procedure and sanction?
  - a complaints mechanism?
- What qualification does the therapist hold?
- What training was involved in getting the qualification(s)?
- How many years has the therapist been practising?
- Is the therapist covered by professional indemnity insurance?

The BMA said that although it would like to see natural therapies regulated by law, with a single regulating body for each therapy, it did not think that all therapies needed regulating. For the majority, it said, 'the adoption of a code of practice, training structures and voluntary registration would be sufficient'.

Complementary Medicine: New Approaches to Good Practice (Oxford University Press, 1993)

Making the choice

The final choice is a matter of using a combination of common sense and intuition and giving someone a try. But do not hesitate to double-check with them when you see them that the information in the listing agrees with what they tell you – nor to cancel an appointment (give at least twenty-four hours' notice if you can) or to walk out if you do not like anything about the person, the place or the treatment. The important advice at all times is to ask questions, as many as you need to, and use your intuition. Never forget: it is your body and mind!

What is it like seeing a natural therapist?

In a word, different. But it is also very natural. Since most therapists, even in those countries with state health systems, still work mainly privately there is no established uniform or common outlook. Though they are all likely to share more or less a belief in the principles outlined in Chapter 7, they represent all walks of life, from the rich to the poor, the politically left to the politically right, and you will come across as much variety in dress, thinking and behaviour as there are fashions, from the elegant and formal to the positively informal and 'woolly-haired' (though, for image reasons, many now wear a white coat to look more like a doctor!).

Equally, you will find their premises very different – reflecting their attitudes to their work and the world. Some will present a 'brass plaque' image, working in a clinic or room away from home with receptionist and brisk efficiency, while others will see you in their living room surrounded by pot plants and domestic clutter. Remember, though, image may be some indication of status but it is little guarantee of ability. You are as likely to find a therapist of quality working from home as in a formal clinic.

There are some characteristics, however, probably the most important ones, you will find common to all natural therapists.

- They will give you far more time than you are used to with a family doctor. An initial consultation will rarely last less than an hour, and often longer. During it they will ask you all about yourself so they can form a proper understanding of what makes you tick and what may be the fundamental cause(s) of your problem.

- They will charge you for their time and for any remedies they prescribe, which they may well sell you themselves from their own stocks. But many therapists offer reduced fees, and even waive fees altogether, for deserving cases or for people who genuinely cannot afford it.

Sensible precautions

- Though most practitioners charge fees no ethical person will ask for fees in advance of treatment unless for special tests or medicines, but even this is unusual. If you are asked for 'down payments' of any sort ask exactly what for and if you don't like the reasons refuse to pay.
- Be sceptical of anyone who 'guarantees' you a cure. No one (not even doctors) can.
- Be very wary of stopping drugs prescribed by your family doctor on the therapist's insistence without first talking things over with your doctor. Non-medical therapists know little about pharmaceutical drugs and there may be danger to yourself if you stop suddenly or without preparation.
- If you are female feel free to have someone with you if you need to undress and if being accompanied makes you feel more comfortable. No ethical therapist will refuse such a request, and if they do, have nothing more to do with them.

What to do if things go wrong

The most important thing to decide is whether you think the therapist has done his or her absolute best to get you better without hurting or harming you in any way. Failure to cure you is not an offence (the truth is, it is probably as much as disappointment to the therapist as it is to you) but failure to take proper care and treat you with professional respect is. If this should happen to you, and you feel it is as the result of behaviour which you regard as either incompetent or unethical, you could consider the following actions.

● If you feel the therapist was doing his or her best to help but simply wasn't good enough it might be as well, for the safety of future patients as much as for the therapist's sake, to talk the problem over with him or her first. He or she may be oblivious of any short-comings and be not only grateful for your constructive honesty but see a way to make amends and help you further.

But if the situation is more serious than this then you have no option but either to turn your back on the whole episode or take further action.

● Report them to their professional association or society if they have one.

(Don't expect this to lead to dramatic changes however. Because unconventional medicine still belongs in many ways to an unestablished, and even sometimes anti-establishment, sub-culture – it has been called 'the folk medicine of the masses' – it exists in many countries still in a sort of unregulated limbo world in which pretty well anything goes and there are few official controls. This can have its advantages of course: the better and more original practitioners can experiment and change direction at will in a way they wouldn't be allowed to do if they were tied up in rules and regulations as doctors are. But it also means there is little or no professional comeback if they don't behave in a way you like or think they should. Even if they belong to a professional organization – and, in Britain at least, no practitioner who is not medically trained has to belong to any organization – those organizations have little or no real power to do anything to a member who breaks the rules. In Britain if they expel someone that person is still free to practise under existing common law provided he or she doesn't break any civil or criminal law.)

- Tell anyone and everyone you come across about your experience, especially the person who recommended the therapist, if this applies, and tell the therapist him or herself you are doing so. (But make sure you are telling the truth: deliberately spreading lies which damage someone's reputation and livelihood is a criminal offence.) Practitioners who get themselves a bad reputation are quickly out of business – and rightly so – and to that extent, at least, they are under pressure to behave professionally, and they know it. Ultimately that is your only guarantee. But it is also the best guarantee.

- In the very worst case, which is always possible though rare, you can resort to the civil or criminal law – that is, you can sue or bring a charge for assault – either through a lawyer or by going direct to the police. Alternatively citizens' rights or advice bureaux may be able to help.

Summary

The reality is that although the opportunity is there, resulting in the occasional tabloid newspaper headline, there are few real crooks or charlatans in natural therapy. Despite the myth, there is little real money in it unless the therapist is very busy – and if he or she is the chances are high it is because he or she is good. In fact you are just as likely to find bad practitioners in orthodox medicine and among the ranks of the so-called 'qualified' as among those who work quietly alone at home with no formal training at all. No one can know everything and no one qualified in anything, including medicine, has to get 100 per cent in their exams to be able to practise. Perfection is an ideal, not a reality, and to err is human.

It is very much for this reason that taking control of your own health is perhaps the single most important lesson underlying the series of books of which this is part. For taking control means taking responsibility for the choices you make, and taking responsibility for choices we now know to be one of the most significant factors in successful treatment, whether of yourself or through the intermediate services of a therapist. No one else but you can decide on a practitioner and no one else but you should decide also if practitioners are any good or not, whether they are a conventional doctor or a natural therapist, or both. You will know very easily, and probably very quickly, if they are any good by the way you feel about them and their therapy and by whether or not you get any better.

If you are not happy about them or your progress the decision is yours as to whether you stay or move on – and continue moving until you find the right therapist for you. But do not despair if you don't find the right person first time, and above all never give up hope. There is almost bound to be the right person for you somewhere and your determination to get well is the best resource you have for finding that person.

Above all, bear in mind that many people before you who have taken this route have not only been helped beyond their most optimistic dreams but have also found a close and trusted helper whom they, and their family, can always turn to in times of trouble – and who may even become a friend for life.

APPENDIX A

Useful organizations

The following listing of organizations is for information only and does not imply any endorsement, nor do the organizations listed necessarily agree with the views expressed in this book.

INTERNATIONAL

International Federation of Practitioners of Natural Therapeutics
46 Pulens Crescent
Sheet
Petersfield
Hampshire GU31 4DH, UK.
Tel 0730 266790
Fax 0730 260058

AUSTRALASIA

Acupuncture Ethics and Standards Organization
PO Box 84
Merrylands
New South Wales 2160.

Arthritis and Rheumatism Foundation of New Zealand
PO Box 10-020
Southern Cross Building
Brandon Street
Wellington
New Zealand.

Australian Arthritis and Rheumatism Foundation
The Queen Elizabeth Hospital
Woodville
South Australia 5011.

Australian Natural Therapists Association
PO Box 308
Melrose Park
South Australia 5039.
Tel 8297 9533
Fax 8297 0003

Australian Traditional Medicine Society
PO Box 442
or
Suite 3, First Floor,
120 Blaxland Road
Ryde
New South Wales 2112.
Australia.
Tel 2808 2825
Fax 2809 7570

International Federation of Aromatherapists
35 Bydown Street
Neutral Bay
New South Wales 2089
Australia

New Zealand Natural Health Practitioners Accreditation Board
PO Box 37-491
Auckland, New Zealand.
Tel 9 625 9966
Supported by 15 therapy organizations.

New Zealand Register of Acupuncturists
PO Box 9950
Wellington 1
New Zealand.

Western Australia Arthritis and Rheumatism Foundation
PO Box 7157
Cloisters Square
Perth 6000
Western Australia.

NORTH AMERICA

American Academy of Medical Preventics
6151 West Century Boulevard
Suite 1114
Los Angeles
California 90045, USA.
Tel 213 645 5350

American Aromatherapy Association
PO Box 3609
Culver City
California 90231

American Association of Acupuncture and Oriental Medicine
National Acupuncture Headquarters
1424 16th Street NW, Suite 501
Washington DC 200 36, USA.

American Association of Naturopathic Physicians
2800 East Madison Street,
Suite 200
Seattle
Washington 98112, USA.
or
PO Box 20386
Seattle
Washington 98102, USA.
Tel 206 323 7610
Fax 206 323 7612

American Holistic Medical Association
4101 Lake Boone Trail
Suite 201
Raleigh
North Carolina 27607, USA.
Tel 919 787 5146
Fax 919 787 4916

Arthritis Foundation
1314 Spring Street
NW
Atlanta
Georgia 30326, USA.

Arthritis Information Clearinghouse
PO Box 34427
Bethesda
Maryland 20034, USA.

Arthritis Society
920 Yonge Street
Suite 420
Toronto
Ontario M4W 3J7, Canada.

**Canadian Holistic Medical
Association**
700 Bay Street
PO Box 101, Suite 604
Toronto
Ontario M5G 1Z6, Canada.
Tel 416 599 0447

**North American Society of
Homoeopaths**
4712 Aldrich Avenue
Minneapolis 55409, USA.

SOUTHERN AFRICA

**South Africa Rheumatism and
Arthritis Association**
Namaqua House
36 Burg Street
Capetown 8001.

**South African Homoeopaths,
Chiropractors and Allied
Professions Board**
PO Box 17055
0027 Groenkloof
South Africa.
Tel 2712 466 455

UNITED KINGDOM

**Arthritis and Rheumatism
Council for Research**
Copeman House
St Mary's Court
St Mary's Gate
Chesterfield
Derbyshire S41 7TD.
Tel 01246 558033.

Arthritis Care
18 Stephenson Way
London NW1 2HD.
Tel 0171 916 1500

**British Complementary
Medicine Association**
St Charles Hospital
Exmoor Street
London W10 6DZ.
Tel 0181 964 1205
Fax 0181 964 1207

**British Holistic Medical
Association**
Royal Shrewsbury Hospital
South
Shrewsbury
Shropshire SY3 8XF.
Tel 01743 261155
Fax 01743 353637

**Council for Complementary and
Alternative Medicine**
179 Gloucester Place
London NW1 6DX.
Tel 0171 724 9103
Fax 0171 724 5330

Disabled Living Foundation
380–384 Harrow Road
London W9 2HU.
Tel 0171 289 6111

Health Education Authority
Hamilton House
Mabledon Place
London WC1H 9TX.
Tel 0171 383 3833
Fax 0171 387 0550

Institute for Complementary Medicine
PO Box 194
London SE16 1QZ.
Tel 0171 237 5165
Fax 0171 237 5175

Royal Association for Disability and Rehabilitation
12 City Forum
250 City Road
London EC1V 8AF.
Tel 0171 250 3222

Yoga for Health Foundation
Ickwell Bury
Biggleswade
Bedfordshire SG18 9EF.
Tel 01767 627271

APPENDIX B

Useful further reading

Acupuncture, Peter Mole (Element Books, UK/USA, 1992)

Classical Homoeopathy, Margery Blackie, ed Charles Elliott and Frank Johnson (Beaconsfield Publishers, UK, 1986)

Conquering Pain, Sampson Lipton (Martin Dunitz, London, 1984)

Information for People with Arthritis (General information booklet published by Arthritis Care, which publishes many other leaflets and booklets. Address in Appendix A)

Introducing Arthritis (General information booklet published by the Arthritis and Rheumatism Council. The council publishes many other leaflets and booklets on various aspects of arthritis and rheumatism. Address in Appendix A)

Is Acupuncture for You?, J R Worsley (Element Books UK/USA, 1985)

Nutritional Medicine, Stephen Davies and Alan Stewart (Pan Books, UK, 1987)

Overcoming Arthritis, Frank Dudley Hart (Positive Health Guide series, Martin Dunitz, London, 1981)

Reader's Digest Family Guide to Alternative Medicine, ed Patrick Pietroni (The Reader's Digest Association, London, New York, Sydney, Montreal, Cape Town, 1991)

Rheumatism and Arthritis, Malcolm Jayson and Allan St J Dixon (Pan Books, London, Sydney and Auckland, 1991)

Understanding Arthritis, Verna Wright (BMA Family Doctor Publications, London, 1993)

Understanding Rheumatism, Frank Dudley Hart (BMA Family Doctor Publications, London, 1986)

Which? Way to Health, The Consumers' Association, (on homoeopathy, October 1992)

Which? Way to Health, The Consumers' Association, (on hypnotherapy, December 1993)

Index